BIOMEDICAL DEVICES AND THEIR APPLICATIONS

NANOPARTICLES AND THEIR CONJUGATES FOR BIOMEDICAL APPLICATIONS

AN ADVANCED MATERIAL FOR DIAGNOSIS AND THERAPEUTIC TREATMENT

BIOMEDICAL DEVICES AND THEIR APPLICATIONS

Additional books and e-books in this series can be found on Nova's website under the Series tab.

BIOMEDICAL DEVICES AND THEIR APPLICATIONS

NANOPARTICLES AND THEIR CONJUGATES FOR BIOMEDICAL APPLICATIONS

AN ADVANCED MATERIAL FOR DIAGNOSIS AND THERAPEUTIC TREATMENT

ANEEYA KUMAR SAMANTARA
AND
SATYAJIT RATHA
EDITORS

nova
Medicine & Health
New York

Library of Congress Cataloging-in-Publication Data

ISBN: 978-1-53616-596-8
Library of Congress Control Number:2019953070

Published by Nova Science Publishers, Inc. † New York

Dr. Aneeya K. Samantara would like to dedicate this work to,
His parents, Mr. Braja Bandhu Dash,
Mrs. Swarna Chandrika Dash and his beloved wife Elina

Dr. Satyajit Ratha would like to dedicate this work to,
His Parents, Mrs. Prabhati Ratha and Mr. Sanjaya Kumar Ratha

Contents

PREFACE

Nanostructured materials, owing to their peculiar surface chemistry and unprecedented physical properties have penetrated to almost every areas pertaining to science, be it catalysis, charge storage, optical, or biological applications. This book encompasses the revolutionary success of nanotechnology and nanostructured materials in revolutionizing the various aspects of pharmaceutics and therapeutics including diagnosis techniques and repair thereof. Though most of the emerging trends in both biological and medical sciences are highly diverse in nature, they cannot be, in anyways, ignored, considering the fact that each one of them would be interlinked and can provide just the required amount of push to address various issues/bottlenecks in the field of diagnosis, therapy, and implantations.

This book introduces some fundamental techniques of fabrication at nanoscale to familiarize the readers with the origin of the nanostructured materials. Furthermore, a brief account of their application has been provided through in a manner so as to explore the diverse nature of these as-prepared nanostructures. Several key aspects of medicinal and therapeutics biology such as bio-sensing, bio-imaging, tissue engineering, nanomedicines including dentistry have been included in this book to explore the next-generation solution through nanotechnology and the subsequent excerpts from the traditional methods to draw a clear cut understanding of the differences (improvements and/or modifications) that have been achieved. Finally, the challenges of mass production and acceptance of nanotechnology by the medical community are considered.

ACRONYMS

µm	micro meter
2D	two dimensions
3D	three dimensions
ACP	amorphous calcium phosphate
ADSC	adipose-derived stem cell
AFM	atomic force microscopy
Ag	Silver
Ag	silver
Al	Aluminum
Al2O3	aluminium oxide
AP	Acute pancreatitis
Au NP	Gold nanoparticle
Au	Gold
BHQ-2	black-hole quencher-2
BMPs	bone morphogenetic proteins
C_{60}	Fullerenes
CAs	contrast agents
Cd	Cadmium
CDs	carbon dots
CeO2	cerium oxide
CFSE	carboxy fluoresceindiacetatesuccinimidyl ester

CHS	Chitosan
CNF	Carbon Nanofiber
CNS	central nervous system
CNS	central nervous system
CNT	carbon nano tubes
CNTs	carbon nanotubes
Co	Cobalt
CQDs	carbon quantum dots
CT	Chemotherapy
CT	computed tomography
CT	computed tomography
CT	Computed Tomography
Cu	Copper
CVD	Chemical vapour deposition
CVD	chemical vapour deposition
DC	direct current
DFI	Diffusion reflection imaging
DLS	Dynamic light scattering
DNA	deoxyribonucleic acid
DTPA	diethyltriaminepentaacetic acid
DTT	dithiothreitol
EC	electrochemical
ECL	electrochemiluminescence
ECM	extracellular matrix
EDC	ethylene dicarbonate
EDTA	ethylene diamines tetra acetic acid
ELISA	Enzyme-linked immunosorbent assay
EPR	Enhanced permeability and retention
FA-PEG-PLGA-NPs	Folate coupled polyethylene glycolylated polylactide-coglycolide nanoparticles
FDA	Food and Drug Administration
Fe	Iron
Fe2O3	Iron oxide

Fe3O4	magnetite
FI	fluorescent imaging
FITC	fluorescent dyes such as fluoresceinisothiocyanate
FRET	Fluorescence resonance electron transfer
gel	continuous liquid phase
GFP	green fluorescent protein
GH	Gadolinium based hybrid
GIC	glass ionomer cement
GMR	magneto resistive
GNPs	Gold nano particles
GNPs	gold nanoparticles
GNPs	gold nanoparticles
GNR	Gold nanorods
GO	Graphene Oxide
GO	graphene oxide
HA	hydroxyapatite
HAp	Hydroxy apatite
HCC	Hepatocellular carcinoma
HIV	human immunodeficiency virus
hMSCs	human mesenchymal stem cells
i.m	intramuscular
i.t.	Intrathecal
i.v	intravenous
IL-6	Interleukin 6
IRIV	immunopotentiating reconstituted influenza virosome
LA	local anaesthetics
LASER	Light Amplification by Stimulated Emission of Radiation
LI	luminescent imaging
LSPR	localized surface plasmon resonance
MAPK	mitogen-activated protein kinase
MAPS	Molecularly activated plasmonic nanosensors
MCLs	magnetite cationic liposomes
MNPs	magnetic nanoparticles
MNPs	Magnetic nanoparticles

MPS	mononuclear phagocytic system
MRI	Magnetic resonance imaging
MRI	magnetic resonance imaging
MRI	Magnetic Resonance Imaging
MSCs	mesenchymal stem cells
MTT	1-(2-mercaptoethyl)-1, 3, 5- triazinane-2, 4, 6-trione
MwCNT	multiwalled carbon nanotubes
NADH	nicotinamide adenosine dinucleotide reduced
Nano-HA	Nano hydroxyapatite
NBs	nanobubbles
nFAp	nano-fluoroapatite
NIR	near Infra-Red
NIR	near infra-red
nm	nanometer
NMR	nuclear magnetic resonance
NPs	Nanoparticles
NPs	Nanoparticles
OCT	Optical coherence tomography
OPMDs	Oral potentially malignant disorders
OSCC	Oral squamous cell carcinoma
OTC	oxytetracycline
PAI	photoacoustic imaging
PANI	Poly aniline
Pb	Lead
PCL	poly(ε-caprolactone)
PCL	polycaprolactone
PCLs	polyacrylates and poly(caprolactone)s
PCR	Polymerase chain reaction
PDDA	Poly (diallyldimethylammonium)
PDGFs	detection of platelet-derived growth factors
PDLSCs	periodontal ligament mesenchymal stem cells
PEG	polyethylene glycol
PEI	Poly ethylene imine
PET	positron emission tomography

PET	positron emission tomography
PGA	polyglycolide
PGC	poly(glycolide-cocaprolactone)
PGLA	Poly lactide-co-glycolide
PL	photo luminescent
PL	photoluminescence
PLA	polylactic acid
PLA	polylactide
PLC	poly(lactide-co-caprolactone)
PLGA	poly (lactide-co-glycolide)
PLGA	poly(lactide-glycolide)
PLLA	poly(L-lactic acid)
PMMA	poly methylmethacrylate
ppb	parts per billion
PPy	poly pyrrole
PU	poly urethane
PVP	poly (vinyl pyrrolidone)
PVP	polyvinylpyrrolidone
QAS-PEI	Quaternary ammonium polyethylenimine
QDs	quantum dots
QDs	Quantum dots
RB	Rose Bengal
RMGIC	Resin modified glass ionomer cement
RNA	Ribose Nucleic Acid
ROS	reactive oxygen species
s.c.	subcutaneous
SCC	Squamous cell carcinoma
SERS	surface enhanced Raman scattering
SERS	Surface-enhanced Raman scattering
SiNPs	silica nanoparticles
SiNPs	Silica nanoparticles
SiO2	silicon dioxide
SNPs	silver nanoparticles
sol	colloidal suspension

SPECT	single photon emission computed tomography
SPECT	single photon emission computed tomography
SPIONs	Super paramagnetic iron oxide NPs
SPR	surface plasmon resonance
TE	Tissue engineering
TEM	Transmission electron microscopy
TEOS	tetraethoxysilanes
TEOS	tetraethylorthosilicate
TiO2	titanium oxide
TMOS	tetramethoxysilane
TMOS	tetramethylorthosilicate
TNF- α	Tumour necrosis factor-alpha
TNT	2, 4, 6-trinitrotoluene
UCL	upconversion luminescence
UCNPs	upconversion nanoparticles
USI	ultrasound imaging
UV	ultra violet
VEGF	vascular endothelial growth factor
VEGF	Vascular endothelial growth factor
Zn	Zinc
ZnO	Zinc oxide

In: Nanoparticles
Editors: A. K. Samantara, S. Ratha
ISBN: 978-1-53616-596-8

Chapter 1

NANOMATERIALS BASED STRATEGIES FOR BIO-SENSING APPLICATIONS

Eepsita Priyadarshini*
School of Environmental Sciences,
Jawaharlal Nehru University, New Delhi, India

ABSTRACT

Nanomaterial based technology has vast implications and opportunities for design and generation of biosensing tools. Metal based nanoparticles and quantum dots have emerged as new generation tools for selective and sensitive detection of analytes such as pesticides, biomolecules, heavy metal ions, DNA and oligonucleotides. Basically, detection and quantification of analytes are limited to the traditional chromatographic and spectrophotometric methods, which are limited by the costly instrumentation, lengthy sample preparation process and on-site contamination. Nanomaterials that include nanoparticles, nanoconjugates, nanocomposites and quantum dots circumvent these limitations by providing a high surface to volume ratio, easy surface accessibility and cost-effectiveness. These nanomaterials facilitate the generation of smart sensors and detection tools for biological entities.

* Corresponding Author's Email: lisa.eepsita@gmail.com.

Biosensor basically refers to an analytical detection device that includes a biological sensor and a physical transducer, wherein the binding of a specific analyte induces the generation of a signal that is measurable. Nanomaterials based sensors provide the advantages of cost-effectiveness, on-site analysis and versatility. In this chapter, a brief overview of the advances in bio-sensing technology using nanomaterials has been presented. Specifically, the applicability of three different kinds of biosensors (optical, fluorescence and electrochemical) has been elaborately discussed. Afterwards, the current state-of-art of nanomaterials for bio-sensing application and the detailed mechanism behind the detection process has been described. The tuneable optical and fluorescence properties of nanoparticles and the effect of surface functionalization have been briefly presented followed by a discussion on the general groups of suitable nanoparticles for the sensing application. The chapter concludes with a discussion on the application of nanostructured particles for sensing of various analytes followed by summary and future perspective.

Keywords: bio-sensing, metal nanoparticles, quantum dots, electro-chemical, colorimetric, fluorescence

1. Introduction

Particles with one or more dimensions in the size range of 1 – 100 nm have been defined as nanoparticles (NPs) by the European Union Commission. Similarly, nanomaterials have been termed as "incidental, natural or manufactured materials existing in an unbound or bound state and where more than 50% particles possess one or more dimensions in the size range of 1 – 100 nm" (Schmid and Andreas 1989, 609). Nanoparticles have been extensively studied due to their promising applicability in various domains such as catalysis, electronics, drug delivery, diagnosis, cancer treatment, therapy and bio-sensing. Amidst these, the use of nanoparticles for bio-sensing application is one of the most active research thrust. A wide range of analytes have been detected using nanomaterials that includes a) nanosensors for disease diagnosis b) nanobio-sensors for environmental applications c) nanobased cell trackers d) nanoprobes for cellular imaging, drug therapy and disease pathway monitoring (Jain 2007,

2002; Jain 2008, 89; Zhao 2011, 490201; Conde 2012, 619530; Baptista 2011, 427). The miniscule size, large surface area and high stability of nanoparticles have made them well-suited candidates for bio-sensing (Azzazy 2009, 1).

A plethora of nanomaterials are being developed and appropriately engineered for devising new protocols of bio-sensing. The properties and subsequent application of nanomaterials basically relies on their size, surface morphology and chemical composition. On basis of properties, we can briefly categorize them into metal nanoparticles, semiconductor based nanomaterials or quantum dots and magnetic nanomaterials. The most common and widely used nano-scaled substrate for bio-sensing includes metal nanoparticles, more specifically gold nanoparticles (GNPs) and silver nanoparticles (SNPs). Metal nanoparticles because of their tuneable optical properties, easy functionalization and aqueous solubility have been significantly used in sensing and detection application (Reddy 2012, 5818; Colombo 2012, 4306). The unique surface plasmon resonance (SPR) property of metal nanoparticles has been significantly used for application in disease diagnosis, bio-imaging, drug delivery, and therapeutics and gene delivery. Quite recently, semiconductor based quantum dots are being investigated for bio-sensing by utilizing the high stability, superior quantum yield and photoluminescence efficiency (Wang 2013, 2786). Several reports postulate the toxic nature of quantum dots that limits their applications in biomedicines. Therefore, new strategies are being developed for functionalizing the quantum dot surface by ligand exchange reactions thereby making the quantum dots non-toxic. Magnetic nanoparticles (MNPs) in particular, iron oxide nanoparticles have also been studied for its bio-sensing application based on super paramagnetism property (Rocha-Santos 2014, 28). MNPs of size 10-20 nm with defined dimension and properties are widely used in disease diagnosis, therapy, cellular imaging and water purification (Ambashta 2010, 38; Perez 2002, 816). The high mass transference along with the size-dependent physicochemical property makes them of wide significance in bio-sensing application. These intriguing properties of nanomaterials assist in augmenting the performance of biosensors by enhancing the selectivity and sensitivity of the system. Thus, these nanoscaled materials have emerged as excellent platforms for design and development of protocols for biosensing application, showing versatility in wide domains from biological to chemical samples. In this chapter, a brief outline of the use of nanoparticles in bio-sensing has been presented. Additionally, the mechanism behind nanoparticles functionalization has been described in details. A categorical analysis of the various types of nanomaterials in bio-sensing and the corresponding mechanism in detection of analytes has also been presented.

2. Functionalization of Nanoparticles

Nanoparticle based application involve interaction of particle surface with the surrounding environment and hence, it's necessary to specifically modify the NP surface to elicit the desired response. For instance, if we are targeting the detection of breast cancer cell lines, we have to modify the surface of NPs with breast cancer markers that would result in specific antigen-antibody (Ag-Ab) reaction, favouring precise identification of specific cells. In contrast, some studies demand non-interaction of NP with the surrounding environment. Figure 1 illustrates a schematic representation of the two different mechanism of detection. In such cases it is necessary to sheath the NP surface with molecules that prevent their interaction/uptake by cellular system. Polyethylene glycol (PEG) is the most commonly used substrate in such cases, which increases the shelf life of NP in blood circulation and enhances the retention time in protein rich solution (Cho 2010, 116; Shyh-Dar and Huang 2011, 178). It's hypothesized that PEG inhibits the formation of protein corona resulting in non-recognization of NP by the host immune system and therefore, PEGlyated NPs are used in most in vitro studies to reduce their uptake by cells compared to their bare counterparts. In addition, the dipolar attraction between nanoparticles surface often leads to their agglomeration in biological rich solutions. In such cases, it is necessary to stabilize the NP surface with surface coating agents that will prevent further growth of particles and render a specific surface charge that minimizes the electrostatic attraction among particles.

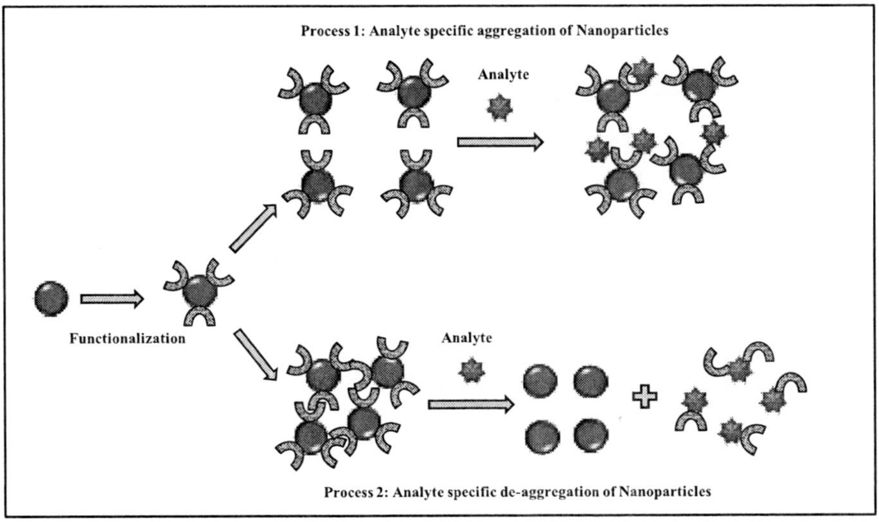

Figure 1. Schematic illustration of the two different mechanisim behind detection of analyte molecules using functionalized nanoparticles.

Thus, functionalization refers to the process of appropriately modifying the surface of NP with surface coating agents or specific ligands/peptide molecules so as to obtain a desired response. In situ synthesis, surface encapsulation and self-assembly are some of the strategies being employed recently to achieve surface functionalization (Priyadarshinhi and Pradhan 2016, 888). The different types of biomolecules used for functionalizing includes synthetic polymers, bio-polymers, peptide molecules, dendrimers and small ligand molecules (Priyadarshinhi and Pradhan 2016, 888). These functionalized NPs represent an important class of substrate in development of miniature sensors because of the high sensitivity and selective response. Such NPs based sensor essentially comprise of two components: recognition moiety (assists in selective binding) and transducer (transmits the signal). Quite recently, GNPs, QDs and MNPs have been vastly used for detection of metal ions, proteins, nuclei acids and other small bio-analytes (Prez 2002,

816). The interaction chemistry of biomolecules and metal NP conjugation can occur via four different mechanisms that include electrostatic interaction, chemisorption, covalent bonding and affinity-based binding (Templeton 2000, 27).

Electrostatic interaction involves the interaction between negative and positive charged groups, for instance adsorption of DNA on positively charged metal NPs. Whereas the chemisorption involves the classical thiol-Au binding (Templeton 2000, 27). As the name suggests affinity based binding involves binding between an affinity pair for example an antigen-antibody interaction, wherein the NP is conjugated with an antibody and the target ligand with Ab-specific antigen molecule (Templeton 2000, 27). NP conjugation with biomolecules like amines, carboxylic acid can also occur via covalent linkage (Sun 2002, 2176; Zrazhevskiy 2010, 4326). In addition, conjugation of biomolecules to QDs is assisted via metal-affinity driven self-assembly process. In a particular work, Medintz et al., 2003 conjugated biomolecules to CdSe/ZnS QDs (Medintz 2003, 630). They have used the polyhistidine tags attached to biomolecule C- and N- terminus which can in turn coordinate with the Zn ions of ZnS coated CdSe QDs. Afterwards, these CdSe/ZnS QDs functionalized with black-hole quencher-2 (BHQ-2) and employed for the detection of DNA. In this case, the detection was based on quenching of QD fluorescence when modified with BHQ-2. However, when the conjugated QDs bind with target DNA, it leads to DNA degradation, removal of BHQ-2 from QD surface thereby leading to an enhancement in fluorescence intensity (Freeman 2011, 4456). In another work, the Texas Red-labeled peptide modified CdSe/ZnS QDs were used to study proteolytic activity by targeting caspase 3, (an effector of cellular apoptosis) (Prasuhn 2010, 5487).

MNPs are normally prone to irreversible aggregation and hence have to be stabilized by appropriate surface coating agents prior to their application. MNPs are generally stabilized by surfactant molecules such as dextran or PEG that form a stabilizing coating on the core (Reddy 2012, 5818). In another study, Fe_3O_4 MNPs modified with prostate-specific membrane Ag aptamer were reported as excellent nanotheranostic agent

(Yu 2011, 2241). Similarly, PEGylated gold nanorods were conjugated with a monoclonal antibody, cetuximab that was in turn used as the ragnostic probes targeting epithelial cancer cells (Choi 2012, 746). Glucose detection sensors were developed using GNPs fabricated with glucose oxidase (Zhang 2005a, 15). Based on these strategies numerous nano-sensors have been designed for selective, rapid and sensitive detection of analyte molecules, which have been described in detail in subsequent sections.

3. Nanomaterials for Biosensing Application

3.1. Metal Nanoparticles

Noble metal based NPs are the most extensively studied class of material that have found applications in catalysis, electronics, pharmaceutical, diagnosis and therapeutics. Numerous physical and chemical methods have been employed for synthesizing noble metal NPs with well-defined size and monodispersity (Khomutov 2002, 141; Oliveira 2005, 429). Homogenous colloidal dispersion of NPs renders them with unique physicochemical properties for sensing and detection application. GNPs are the most sought-after material for bio-sensing application due to their distinctive optical property and easy surface modulation ability (Boisselier 2009, 1759). GNPs are synthesized basically by chemical reduction wherein Au^{3+}gets reduced to Au^{0} state using a reducing agent. The classical Turkevich method uses sodium citrate as the reducing and capping agent, generating GNPs in the range of 5 – 20 nm size which was stabilized by electrostatic repulsion between individual particles (Turkevich 1954, 26). Number of alternative synthesis protocols using aqueous and organic solvents has been explored to achieve controlled size and shape of particles. Moreover, studies are focusing on understanding the chemistry of synthesis and functionalization with different biomolecules so as to generate engineered NPs for bio-sensing application. Noble metal NPs have been explored for detection of a range of bio-molecules including nucleic acids, proteins, enzymes and metal ions based on the unique surface plasmon resonance phenomenon. SPR, fluorescence quenching, electrochemical and surface enhanced Raman scattering (SERS) properties, SPR is the most commonly used phenomenon in bio-sensing due to the simplicity, ease of the process, portability and eco-friendless that allows the development of point-of-care devices. Mostly, silver and gold nanoparticles due to their unique SPR property, ease of synthesis and modification have been widely used in biosensing application. The detailed mechanism behind the SPR based or colorimetric mode of detection has been described in the following section.

3.2. Quantum Dots

Quantum dots (QDs) represent a unique class of fluorescent nanomaterials synthesized usually from semiconductor crystals belonging to group II and VI elements of periodic table. Some of the common examples of QDs include CdSe, CdTe, InAs and ZnSe particles. QDs have become increasing important as imaging and detection probes due to their high stability, superior fluorescence quantum yield, large molar extinction coefficient and wide photoluminescence ranging from UV to near infrared region (Dabbousi 1997, 9463). Additionally, QDs are quite stable to photo bleaching and hence have been widely exploited in in vivo bio-imaging. Moreover, they offer tunability of optical properties by varying the size and chemical composition. Another superior feature offered by QDs is their potential to be excited at a single wavelength due to the broad absorbance but narrow emission (Regulacio 2010, 621; Zhong 2003, 8589). QD based biological applications basically require their conjugation with a hydrophilic surface coating ligand. This is due to the fact that fluorescent QDs are generally synthesized in organic solvent via hydrothermal reaction or reverse micelle method (Liu 2013, 15015; Hosseini 2015, 51). The QD surfaces are capped with hydrophobic long chain alkyl amines/carboxyl groups or with oleylamines. It is therefore essential to modify the surface of QDs with proteins, peptides or antibodies to render them biocompatible and aqueous soluble (Tholouli 2008, 275). Surface modification of QDs is essential so as to allow the participation of the particles in the biological environment and thereby generate potent probes for bio-imaging, cellular tracking, therapeutics and bio-sensing (Ho 2010, 60; Dubertret 2002, 1759).

3.3. Carbon Dots

Carbon dots (CDs) also belong to the group of fluorescent semiconductor QDs however, are rich in carbon moieties as they are synthesized by catalytic reduction of carbon-rich compounds. Photoluminescence, tunable optical properties and biocompatibility are the superior features of carbon dots that have made them of significant interest recently (Li 2012, 24230). There has been an exponential rise in studies involving the synthesis and fabrication of CDs since last few years (Li 2012, 24230). As CDs allow easy surface modulation and their fluorescent properties can be modulated by functionalization or doping they are being extensively analysed for potent biomedical applications, specifically in bio-sensing and as bio-imaging probes (Wang 2014, 6921; Lim 2015, 362). Li et al., 2010 synthesized CDs via electrochemical process by using graphite rods and NaOH/ethanol as electrolyte solution (Li 2010, 4430). On fractionation, they observed blue, green, yellow and orange coloured emission on basis of their size and no change in luminescence was found when treated with hydrogen plasma thus suggesting that luminescence property comes from the CDs and not the carbon-oxygen groups. The luminescence property varies when synthesized by chemical process. CDs synthesized by oxidizing graphite oxide using nitric acid and sodium borohydride showed a shift in the emission maxima from 520 to 450 nm respectively. An increase in quantum yield from 2% to 24% was also observed (Zheng 2011, 10650). Additionally, pH and the solvent medium also affect the quantum yield of CDs (Pan 2010, 3681) however; the exact mechanism behind CD luminescence is not completely understood.

3.4. Magnetic Nanoparticles

Quite recently, there has been extensive interest in synthesis of magnetic nanoparticles due to their size, interesting physico-chemical properties and low production cost (Wu 2015, 023501). As it is well known that the properties of MNPs depend on its size and morphological dimensions, it is essential to define the synthesis process appropriately so as to generate particles with efficient physicochemical properties. A number of MNPs have been synthesized that includes iron oxides, iron-platinum particles, iron-cobalt particles, manganese oxide nanoparticles as well as composites of iron oxide nanoparticles (Wu 2015, 023501). Magnetic nanoparticles are basically synthesized by physical or chemical modes. Gas-phase deposition and lithography are the two major physical means of synthesizing MNPs. In addition, sol-gel synthesis, oxidation, co-precipitation, vapour-phase and thermal deposition are some the widely used chemical means for generation of MNPs (Akbarzadeh 2012, 1; Reddy 2012, 5818). However, physical means suffers from the disadvantages of controlled synthesis, which instigated researchers towards microbial mode of synthesis. Moreover, microbial mode offers the superiority of eco-friendliness, low cost, stability and high yield (Beveridge 2011, 251).

As already discussed, properties of NPs depend on their size and morphology. Likewise, the size and shape of MNPs determine their corresponding physico-chemical properties. Due to the small size of MNPs, they are super paramagnetic and hence have a neutral dipole moment. The magnetic nature of particles depends on a number of factors including the crystalline nature, property of starting material and spin number. Because of the super paramagnetic nature, at very high temperature and zero electromagnetic field, MNP do not possess any magnetic moment. On application of a magnetic field a dipole moment is generated and MNPs orient themselves in random directions and return to their original native state alignment after removal of the external electromagnetic field. A magnetometer is generally used for monitoring the magnetism of a material on application of external magnetic field (Li 2010, 4430). This super paramagnetic nature of MNPs makes them superior alternatives in bio-sensing compared to their non-magnetic counterparts. There are two basic strategies in MNP based sensing, in the first case the MNP sensor is incorporated into the transducer material while on the other hand MNPs are dispersed in the sample solution and an external magnetic field is applied at the surface of the material. MNPs based sensors offer several advantages such as high sensitivity with a very low detection limit, shorter detection time and high signal/noise ratio (Justino 2013, 27). Amongst MNPs, Fe_3O_4 NPs are most widely used in bio-sensing application. In addition to their superior super paramagnetic property, feasible synthesis mode, biocompatibility and ease of binding to antibodies/enzyme molecules, they are vastly suitable in sensing applications.

Additionally, MNPs have also been used for development of magneto resistive (GMR) devices. In such devices the signal response is measured in the co-presence of an external magnetic field and hence further decreases the sensitivity of the system, as minute changes in the system can be detected by the generated magnetic field (Sun 2012, 46). The substrates for design of GMR sensors should be monodispersed with high magnetic moment and should be stable in biological solutions (Sun 2012, 46). Li et al., used GMR device approach for detection of interleukin-6, based on the generation of dipole field in response Ab-Ag interaction (Li 2010, 4388). They used two different approaches for interleukin-6 detection. In the first approach, the sensor or MNPs was modified with antibody molecules while in the second approach analyte was conjugated with MNPs. The super paramagnetic nature of MNPs allows their use in development of microfluidic devices that can respond to non-uniform magnetic fields. Such microfluidic system was analyzed for the detection of breast cancer cells wherein it measured the magnetic moments as the MNP conjugated cells flow through the microfluidic device (Issadore 2012, 1). However, MNPs are not quite useful when it comes to multi-analyte detection as magnetic sensors rely on generation of signals from magnetic moment which is a single parameter. For multi-analyte detection, MNPs of varied size and chemical composition will be required that would generate individual non-magnetization curves in response to signals generated upon analyte binding (Issadore 2012, 1).

4. Mechanism of Biosensing

A wide diversity of biosensors have been developed using NPs and QDs for detection of biomolecules and analytes. Most of the detection principle is based on the physico-chemical properties of NPs/QDs and can be broadly categorized into optical sensors and electrochemical sensors. Optical sensors have been greatly explored and used for detection of numerous analytes. They are associated with the advantages of less interference, minimal cost and lower signal-to-noise ratio, which have made them of great interest in clinical, food, environmental and pharmaceutical industries. These optical sensors can be grouped under: localized surface plasmon resonance (LSPR)/colorimetric detection based on property of noble metal NPs & fluorescence based detection using QDs. Similarly, electrochemical sensors based on nanoparticles serve an integral part of biosensing. In this, the electrodes are generally coated with or formed using metal oxide nanoparticles or semiconductors that subsequently serve as the transducer. These nanomaterials are immobilized on the surface of electrode by means of adsorption, covalent bonding or electro deposition. Such modification of electrode allows specific detection of analytes along with the advantages of low cost, sensitivity and portability (Ronkainen 2010, 1747). (The subsequent sub-sections describe in details the mechanism underlying the detection protocol.

4.1. Colorimetric Sensing

Most of the colorimetric based sensors utilize noble metal NPs, specifically silver and gold nanoparticles. These noble metal NPs present distinctive optical properties and ease of functionalization. They present a unique phenomenon termed as LSPR (Localised Surface Plasmon

Resonance) that arises on irradiating the metal surface with electromagnetic waves of suitable wavelength. During the irradiation, collective oscillation of the conduction band electrons takes place on the metal surface leading to the absorption and scattering of the electrons. For noble metal NPs, this property occurs in the UV-visible wavelength range thereby allowing them to be excellent substrates for colorimetric based sensing platforms (Wilcoxon 2009, 2647). Furthermore, size, shape and chemical composition of this nanostructured particle plays a pivotal role in their LSPR property i.e., on increasing the particle size; a red shift (hyperchromic) in the absorption maxima takes place whereasa blue shift occurs on reducing particle size (hypochromic) (Liz-Marzan 2006, 32).

For instance, spherical GNPs in the size range of 10-20 nm show absorption maxima at around 520 nm and are light pink or reddish in colour (Haiss 2007, 4215). But on aggregation, a decrease in the inter-particle distance takes placeleading to an evident change in colour and is reflected in the LSPR band that appears at a longer wavelength region. Colorimetric sensors are thus developed based on this phenomenon of change in colour and shifting of LSPR band on aggregation. The interaction of functionalized GNPs with target analyte leads to the agglomeration of particles and corresponding changes in the optical properties which is used as the basis of detection. Thus, functionalizing NPs with target specific ligands confers high selectivity and renders high sensitive detection. In yet other cases, colorimetric detection is based on the non-specific interaction between bare GNPs and the biomolecules (Li 2011, 817). This mechanism thus makes use of un-functionalized NPs. GNPs have been used as sensor for detection of DNA molecule based on the differential interaction of single stranded DNA (ssDNA) and double stranded DNA (dsDNA). The ssDNA molecules bind with the negatively charged citrate capped GNPs thereby providing an enhanced stability, while the dsDNA do not interact much with the GNPs leading to aggregation of particles on increasing ionic strength. This property has been used for detection of carcinogenic DNA dimers, RNA of hepatitis C virus, nuclei acid, proteins and inorganic ions etc. (Kim 2011, 2805; Shawky 2010, 1163; Xia 2010, 10837). Thiourea and melamine detection has also been achieved using un-functionalized citrate capped GNPs, which aggregate on destabilization of NP surface charge (Wang 2011, 5256; Wei 2010, 133702).

4.2. Fluorescence Sensing

Quantum dots/semiconductor nanocrystals display high photoluminescence (PL) and enhanced stability which has made them promising tools in sensing and bio-imaging. The PL property of QDs is based on the following principle: When a semiconductor QD adsorbs photon, excitation of electrons occurs. This excited electron tends to relax and comes back to ground state leading to the creation of electron-hole and release of electromagnetic energy in the UV to near IR range. Changes in the electron and hole confinement alters the property of the QD. Therefore, QDs exhibit variation in optical properties with change in size and shape of crystal. With decreasing size of QD, the colour shifts from red to blue range of emission light. This property of quantum confinement of QDs plays an integral role in bio-sensing and imaging applications.

Till date, QDs are mostly synthesized using cadmium (Cd), a potentially toxic heavy metal. Reports suggest high level of toxicity from Cd based QDs both from *in vitro* and *in vivo* studies, which are basically due to the degradation of Cd-based QDs in the cellular fluids (Derfus 2004, 11). The correspondingly generated Cd ions, interact with biomolecules resulting in alterations in mitochondrial activity and cellular functioning. Researchers are therefore focusing on synthesis of QDs using non-toxic metal ions or developing strategies towards surface functionalization of CdSe QDs to passivate the toxic Cd core. This would prevent the leakage of the ions into the surrounding medium. In an *in vitro* study, it was deduced that glutathione capped CdSe QDs and ZnS shell encapsulated GSH-CdSe showed a marked reduction in the toxicity of QDs (Kuzyniak 2014, 382). Quite recently, noble metal NPs and QD conjugates have also been investigated for development of fluorescence sensors based on quenching of fluorescence intensity (Priyadarshini 2017, 5425). In some studies, fluorescence property has been combined with magnetic NPs in order to enhance the detection signal. In a particular work, *E.coli* was detected by modifying antigen bound Fe_3O_4 NPs. An external magnetic field was applied that resulted in a reverse magnetic flow leading to the increase in antigen retention time and corresponding rise in the fluorescence signals (Agrawal 2014, 66). One of the basic assay means using QDs involves the direct conjugation of target molecule with QDs. These target molecules can be cells, antibodies or other small biomolecules, which are allowed to interact with the QDs and the resultant unbound QDs are washed from the solution. Thus, the photoluminescence signal generated arises only from the QDs bound to the target analyte (Bruchez 1998, 2013). Another basic mechanism involved QD based sensing is Fluorescence resonance electron transfer (FRET). In this, a fluorophore is attached to the target molecule and relies on the close proximity of donor acceptor pair. The fluorescent molecule serves as the energy acceptor, thereby getting excited and in the process releases light while relaxing to ground state. This mechanism has been widely used for detection of maltose, TNT, cocaine and so on (Goldman 2005, 6744; Zhang 2009, 3051).

4.3. Electrochemical Sensing

This specific category of sensing uses an electrochemical (EC) device to measure the generated signals. In this the electrode surface is basically coated with nanomaterials and when the target analyte interacts with the electrode surface, electrochemical signals in form of current, voltage and impedance is generated which in turn measured by a detector (Xu 2012, 62; Duarte 2014, 21). The working electrode in an EC device can be coated with target specific antibodies, enzymes, nuclei acid molecules or specific recognition molecules (Duarte 2014, 21). Recently nanomaterials are being widely used due to their selectivity and the ability to amplify the signal by several folds. Based on the working mechanism, the EC sensors have been categorized into amperometric, voltammetric, potentiometric or capacitive

(Duarte 2014, 21). EC devices offer several advantages of rapid detection, superior sensitivity, better selectivity, miniaturization and low cost thus making them useful in environmental, clinical and biomedical applications (Duarte 2014, 21). A well-defined EC based immunosensor was reported for detection of ochratoxin-A using iron oxide NPs (Zamfir 2011, 178). In this particular study, the electrode was coated with iron oxide NPs conjugated with antiochratoxin-A monoclonal antibody which offered an enhanced sensitivity. The use of modified NPs decreased the current impedance and allowed reusability by removing the coated NPs and recoating with newly synthesized NPs (Zamfir 2011, 178).

Recently, electrochemiluminescence (ECL) detection has also emerged that uses nanocomposite material. These nanocomposites are synthesized using a combination of magnetic and metal nanoparticles and/or magnetic and quantum dots and/or metal nanoparticles and quantum dots. The use of quantum dots in ECL sensors offers the advantages of high quantum yield and quantum confinement thus offering improved sensitivity (Muzyka 2014, 393). ECL sensors can be developed by relying on direct interaction, competitive interaction or sandwich assay method (Zhou 2012, 107). The combination of MNPs and QDs has been widely investigated as ECL probes. In a classical example, Zhou et al., in the year 2012 have reported a sandwich ECL immunosensor that used MNPs as the capture probes and QDs as the signaling molecules for detection of α-fetoprotein (AFP) (Zhou 2012, 107). In the process, Fe_3O_4-Au NPs were first modified with antibody-1 and CdS-Au particles were modified with antibody 2. When AFP antigen was added to the solution of modified Fe_3O_4-Au NPs, the AFP molecules bind to the antibody site of NPs. Next the free antibody-2 site of CdS-Au NPs binds to the free AFP sites thereby resulting in the construction of Fe_3O_4-Au-A1-AFP-A2-CdS-Au ECL immunosensor. This sandwich system was observed to show enhanced signals compared to the control sets of Fe_3O_4 MNP and CdS QDs. Moreover, the Au moiety here enhanced the signal by 2.5 folds due to the inherent catalytic nature of GNPs. The developed ECL biosensor showed a very high sensitivity comparable to Enzyme Linked Immunosorbent Assay (ELISA and hence can be used in clinical applications.

5. Biosensing Application of Nanoparticles

5.1. Heavy Metal Detection

Heavy metals (Hg, Pb, Cd, As) are known to be quite toxic and pose deleterious effect on human health. Colorimetric sensors have been widely explored for detection of these metal ions in aqueous samples (Priyadarshini 2016, 888). Most of these sensors are based on GNPs which the advantages of functionality and sensitivity. In one such report, DNAzyme- GNPs were utilized for detection of Pb^{2+} ions. DNAzyme gets activated in co-presence of Pb^{2+} leading to the disintegration of GNP aggregates resulting in change in colour of solution which can be easily monitored spectrophotometrically (Liu 2003, 6642). In yet other studies, the colorimetric detection was based on the aggregation of GNPs with a correspondingly red shifting of SPR peak. Based on ion-chelation mechanism the approach was successful in detecting Pb, Cd and Hg ions in aqueous solution (Kim 2001, 165). Cysteine modified GNPs were coated on specifically designed electrodes and used for high specific detection of Cu^{2+} ions and a detection limit of 1 pm was achieved (Gooding 2009, 2015). GNPs functionalized with 11-mercaptoundecanoic acid were used for colorimetric sensing of Pb^{2+}, Cd^{2+}, and Hg^{2+} ions. The specified metal ions induce aggregation of GNPs by chelation with the free carboxylate groups on metal surface. This results in change in colour of solution from red to blue in presence of metal ions (Huang 2007, 1215). Modulation of buffer composition and structure of particle enhanced the sensitivity to 100 nM. The DNA functionalized GNPs have also been used for detection of Hg^{2+} ions. The system is based on thymidine-Hg^{2+}-thymidine coordination and relies on the melting temperature of DNA functionalized GNPs (Liu 2010, 9606). 3-Mercaptopropionate acid and adenosine monophosphate functionalized GNPs have been used for detecting Hg^{2+} ions in aqueous solution. The functionalized GNPs are quite stable and well-dispersed because of efficient electrostatic repulsion between individual particles. Hg^{2+} interacts with the free –COOH groups of MPA leading to the destabilization of surface activity thereby destabilizing GNP assisted by corresponding shift of SPR peak from 520 to 620 nm (Yu 2008, 12717). GNPs functionalized with glutathione, dithiothreitol (DTT) and cysteine were investigated for their ability to detect As^{3+}. The detection limit was in the order of DTT<GSH<Cys, the high affinity of DTT-GNPs towards As^{3+} is because of the high affinity As-S linkage compared to the As-O bonds in case of GSH and Cys functionalization (Kalluri 2009, 1). Similarly, aptamer based colorimetric detection of As^{3+} has also been studied. GNPs were functionalized with Poly (diallyldimethylammonium) (PDDA) and an As^{3+} aptamer. GNPs tend to aggregate in the presence of PDDA, so in presence of As^{3+} ions, aptamer binds to the As^{3+} ions, thereby PDDA molecule are free to bind with GNPs and induce aggregation. In the absence of As^{3+} ions, aptamer and PDDA, a duplex structure was formed that prevents the GNP aggregation forming the basis of detection (Wu 2012, 4459). Similarly, fluorescent nature of CDs has been used for detection of several metal ions. CDs synthesized using citric acid and poly-ethylenimine were used for detection of Cu^{2+} ions (Dong 2012, 6220). The as-synthezised CDs had a quantum yield of 42.5% that was quenched on treatment with Cu^{2+} ions. Basically the Cu^{2+} ions coordinated with the free amine groups available on the CD surface resulting in quenching of fluorescence (Dong 2012, 6220). Detection of Cu^{2+} ions has also been achieved by measuring ratiometric fluorescence intensity of CDs and CdSe/ZnS QDs. The synthesized particle showed an emission at 485 nm and 644 nm due to the CD and CdSe/ZnS counterpart respectively, with the emission at 485 nm being more intense. Thus a blue fluorescence was observed on excitation. However the of Cu^{2+} ions, quenching in the emission signal at 485 nm occurred due to the binding of Cu^{2+} ions to CD surface. Hence, there is a decrease in blue fluorescence intensity leading to corresponding pink colour (Zhu 2012, 7185). In order to further enhance the detection limit, the same group studied an electrochemical basis of Cu^{2+} ions detection, wherein they immobilized the functionalized CDs on an electrode resulting in a detection limit of 100 nM (Shao 2013, 418). Likewise, CDs synthesized form pomelo peel has been reported as excellent Hg^{2+} ion sensors (Lu 2012, 5351). As-synthesized CDs have also been used for fluorescence based detection of Fe^{3+} ion (Xu 2015, 542).

Similarly, CDs synthesized by solid –phase synthesis, with a high quantum yield of 31% was found to quench on addition of Fe^{3+} ions assisted by non-radiative electron transfer (Zhang 2014, 9846). Superoxide anion (O_2^-) was detected using the CDs based on ratiometric fluorescence. It shows a green fluorescence with emission at 525 nm which on interaction with changed to red fluorescence with emission signal at 610 nm (Gao 2014, 7071). A number of metal ions have been detected using CDs based on the fluorescence quenching approach. The fluorescence on-off switch mechanism was used for visible detection of phosphate using Eu^{3+} and aminoundecanoic acid. CDs aggregate by co-ordination between Eu^{3+} ions and carboxylate groups of functional CDs resulting in decreased fluorescence. When phosphate is added to the suspension, Eu^{3+} ions co-ordinate with CDs resulting in re-dispersion. This leads to correspondingly enhanced fluorescence intensity and the defined protocol achieved a detection limit of 51 nM in the linear range of 0.4 – 15 nM (Li 2015, 1922). Similar theories have been used for detection of several metal ions like Co, Mn, Mg, Zn and Ni (Yu 2018).

5.2. Bioanalyte Detection

Besides heavy metals, colorimetric sensing has been demonstrated for detection of bioanalytes. For example, Kim et al., 2010 reported the detection of oxytetracycline (OTC) using aptamer-GNP. The sensor was able to efficiently discriminate OTC among other tetracyclines up to a minimum concentration of 25 nM (Kim 2010, 1644). Sun et al., 2011demonstrated a label free detector for organophosphates using lipoic acid-GNPs based on the acetylcholine esterase activity. The sensor was able to detect organophosphate in pesticides and nerve agents up to picomolar limit (Sun 2011, 152). Similarly, GNPs functionalized with 1-(2-mercaptoethyl)-1, 3, 5- triazinane-2, 4, 6-trione (MTT) were used for sensing of melamine in raw milk. Melamine interacts with MTT via formation of hydrogen bonds resulting in the aggregation of GNPs which forms the basis of detection. A detection limit of 2.5 ppb was achieved by naked eyes within a minute of adding melamine (Ai 2011, 9496). Additionally, thrombin protein present in blood plasma is detected by using GNPs up to pM concentration. The addition of GNP in excess of fibrinogen induces aggregation of fibrin-GNP. By determining the optical density of the resultant supernatant thrombin concentration in plasma can be determined. The sensor developed on basis of this showed an excellent selectivity with a detection range of 0.1 to 10 pM (Chen 2010, 1922). An aptamer-NP strip based sensor was reported for detection of cancer cells which allowed a detection limit of 4000 Ramos cells via naked eyes and 800 Ramos cells via the developed strip reader (Liu 2009, 10013).

Functionalized as well as label-free CDs and QDs have been used for biomolecule sensing. CD based colorimetric sensor has been developed for detecting glucose. The CDs were formed from candle soot and showed peroxidise like activity that assisted in recognition of glucose (Shi 2011, 6695). In one such example, Qian et al., 2015 reported the use of as-synthesized CDs in detection of alkaline phosphatase based on the fluorescence on-off switch (Qian 2015, 2966). Similarly, terbium conjugated CDs were used for ratiometric sensing of dipicolinic acid (Chen 2015, 5036). Ascorbic acid from rat brain was detected using CDs and cobaltoxyhydroxide nanoflakes, wherein the Co nanoflakes served in recognizing ascorbic acid and CDs as the signal generating molecule. Ascorbic acid on interaction with the nanoflakes resulted in its reduction to Co^{2+} ions resulting in the detachment of nanoflakes from the CDs. This was marked by an increase in fluorescence signal (Li 2015, 3404). Specifically boronic acid conjugated CDs were used for sensing of glucose in blood based on the selective interaction of boronic acid with glucose. This interaction resulted in the aggregation of CDs leading to quenching of fluorescence (Lin 2015, 3183). Further, the electrochemiluminescence property of nanomaterials has been used for development of sensors. In one such study, an electrochemical sensor was developed using CDs and chitosan for detection of dopamine (Huang 2013, 5417). Similarly, an electrochemical immunosensor has been reported for α-fetoprotein based on CDs (Dai 2012, 3055). An enzyme based colorimetric biosensor was developed for glucose sensing using modified GNP electrode. Both cyclic voltammetry and electrochemical impedance analysis was performed to analyze the detection limit of the sensor. The sensor showed a limit of 8.2 μM (Zhang 2005b, 826).

5.3. Pesticide and Polluting Agent Detection

Surface plasmon resonance (SPR) principle has been greatly used for development of biosensors. SPR mechanism has been used for detection of huge number of environmental contaminates such as dichloro diphenyl trichloroethane (DDT), atrazine, TNT, biphenyls, carbaryl and so on. In a particular case, the SPR assay technique was used for determination of benzo (a) pyrene, a carcinogenic pollutant that directly correlates with the concentration of polycyclic hydrocarbons in the environment with a detection limit of 10 ppt (Shankaran 2007, 7187). A portable SPR detector was used for determination of carbaryl, DDT and chlorpyrifos. The developed instrument was quite reproducible with a regeneration ability of more than 250 cycles (Mauriz 2007, 1449). In one such approach, CdTe QDs were used as fluorescence probe for detection of monocrotophos. The study involved layer-by-layer assembly of chitosan-CdTe-acetylcholinesterase onto a quartz substrate. Acetylcholine gets hydrolyzed to choline and acetic acid in the absence of pesticide. Production of acetic acid results in decrease in pH which is detected by CdTe, which acts as the pH indicator in this very approach. The fluorescence intensity thus has a direct correlation with concentration of pesticide (Sun 2011, 616).

On basis of the optical property of GNPs, a few pesticide detecting biosensors have been developed. Based on the aggregation of GNPs and the corresponding shift in the SPR peak, organophosphate, diethyl chlorophosphate have been detected up to micromolar concentration. The GNPs in presence of organophosphate showed a blue shift in SPR peak that formed the basis of detection (Newman 2007, 3448). 2,4,6-trinitrotoluene (TNT) is most explosive nitroaromatic compound and is one of the most common contaminating in soil and water samples. GNPs functionalized with cysteine have been used for detection of TNT up to a limit of 2 ppm. The approach is based on the aggregation of GNPs in presence of TNT resulting in a change in colour and shift in SPR peak [109]. GNP-$CaCO_3$ conjugated with acetylcholinesterase was used for electrochemical sensing of organophosphates in water. The detection was quite rapid (<10 sec.) and was based on the inhibition of acetylcholine-esterase by organophosphate and showed a detection limit of 0.1 nm (Chauhan 2011, 923). A highly stable and sensitive electrochemical detector was devised for detection of trichlorfon by using PVP-capped CdS QDs. The detection was based on the enzymatic conversion of trichlorfon to thiocholine with a detection limit of 4.8×10^{-8} M (Li 2006, 2163). Similarly, GNPs have also been used as electrochemical detectors for monocrotophos, carbaryl and methyl parathion. The Au NPs were embedded in a conductive silicate network that favored transfer of electrons and the developed sensor showed a good stability and high storage time of around 30 days (Du 2008a, 766). Additionally, GNPs in combination with QDs have also been reported for detection of monocrotophos, an organophosphorus insecticide. The study showed that the electrochemical sensor formed in combination of CdTe QDs and GNPs was far more sensitive compared to QDs and GNPs alone (Du 2008b, 475). Reports also state the detection of atrazine by using nanoparticles ligated with specific antibodies via competitive interactions. In this, GNPs were labeled with antibodies, coated on electrode surface. Interaction of antigen was recorded by DC measurement resulting in development of a low cost fabricated electrode (Valera 2008, 95). Liu et al., 2006a devised a sensitive electrode for detection of nitrobenze. They conjugated GNPs to multiwall and single-wall carbon nanotubes resulting in a highly sensitive electrode system that was quite responsive to minute changes and achieved a detection limit of 0.3 mg/l (Liu 2006, 139).

5.4. DNA and Oligonucleotide Detection

There has been great interest in detection of DNA and oligonucleotide detection because of their applications in medical technology as in pathogen detection, drug and food industry. Metal nanoparticles, specifically GNPs have dominated this domain of detection as they have demonstrated their potential ability in nucleic acid detection based on aggregation-induced optical variations. Mostly, DNA and aptamer specific probes are used in detection as they hybridize with the target analyte sequence and therefore using functionalized nanoparticles is a necessity in such sensing.To date back, Alivisatos et al., and Elghanian et al., had been the pioneers in colorimetric detection of DNA molecules (Alivisatos 1996, 609; Elghanian 1997, 1078). The classical gold-thiol affinity was used for functionalizing GNP with two different oligonucleotides, complementary to the target DNA sequence. Thus, under appropriate conditions, the DNA molecule can bind with the complementary oligonucleotides thereby dragging the GNPs together resulting in aggregation and subsequent red spectral shift. Based on a similar approach, a "spot-and-read" colorimetric detection protocol was reported that was able to detect 0.3 pM concentration of genomic DNA sample (Storhoff 2004, 883). However, a major limitation of Storhoff et al., process was functionalization of GNPs required 72 hours wherein the GNPs were treated with gradually increasing NaCl concentration. As a solution to this limitation, a negatively charged ligand, BSPP was used, having higher binding affinity towards Au at high salt concentration compared to the classical Au-SH binding affinity (Loweth 1999, 1808; Schmid 1994). This detection limit was brought down to 0.1 pM concentration by fluorescence spectrometric technique based on measuring the changes in resonance light scattering intensity of formed GNP aggregates (Du 2006, 8022). Dynamic light scattering (DLS) has also been used for detection of genomic DNA up to 1 pM concentration (Dai 2008, 8138), but the approach suffers from the disadvantages of requiring large sample amount to allow detection. In yet another study, single molecule biosensing approach was used for genomic DNA detection. This novel approach was based on colour differentiation of individual plasmonic NP, Au/Ag/Au nanocomposite NP and aggregated NPs induced by DNA hybridization. The method detects upto a detection limit of 0.02 pM (Xiao 2010, 6308). Effective GNP based adenosine detectors have been established based on aptazyme based GNP assembly.

Liu et al., constructed an adenosine specific apatamer possessing DNAzyme like activity. The aptazyme remains inactive in absence of adenosine and hence substrate strands act as linker for assembling the DNA conjugated GNPs. In presence of adenosine, aptazyme cleaves substrate strand thereby disrupting the functionalized GNP aggregate (Liu 2006b, 90). In yet another study, aptamer functionalized GNPs were used for detection of platelet-derived growth factors (PDGFs). The detection was based on determination of change in color upon aggregation of functionalized GNPs on addition of PDGFs. The colour changed from red to purple at PDGFs concentration below 400 nM (Huang 2005, 5735). SPR biosensor has been developed for detection of genetically modified organism based on DNA hybridization between the ssDNA probe and the complementary sequence. The sensor involved the immobilization of the DNA probe on SPR sensor (Mariotti 2002, 165). GNPs and dehydrogenase enzyme were used for devising an electrochemical sensor. For this GNPs were assembled on silica with free thiol terminals, which acts as an electrode system. In presence of NADH, the electrode system catalyzes its oxidation thereby decreasing the potential. The system showed a detection limit of 5 nM with a high sensitivity and superior stability (Jena and Raj 2006, 6332).

The classical FRET based mechanism has also been utilized for development of QDs based DNA sensor. In one such study, target DNA was mixed with biotin-DNA probe and Cy5 fluorophore reporter probe. On addition of streptavidin conjugated QDs, a complex (QD-biotin DNA probe-DNA target-Cy5 fluorophore probe) is formed. Thus in the presence of target DNA sequence, the excited light is transferred from the QDs to the reporter probe which was detected by use of a confocal spectroscope (Zhang 2005b, 826). Similar strategies have been used for detection of cocaine, maltose and TNT (Medintz 2003, 630; Goldman 2005, 6744; Zhang 2009, 3051).

SUMMARY AND FUTURE OUTLOOK

In summary, surface engineered and stable nanomaterials have become promising substrates for bio-sensing and effectively complement conventional based sensing applications. Large surface to volume ratio, functionalization, superior optical, chemical and magnetic properties along with plasmonic/fluorescence efficiency of particles offer advantages in biosensing. These specific properties along with property of modulation allow an enhancement in the detection limit with high sensitivity and selectivity of detection. Thus, appropriately functionalized nanomaterials have been significantly used for detection of proteins, nucleic acid, heavy metals and pesticides. Additionally, nanoparticles offer the advantages of generating miniature sensors that allows high throughput analysis with rapidity. It is thus envisaged that by appropriately controlling the physico-chemical properties and incorporation of multifunctionalilty, simultaneous detection of multiple analytes/biomolecules can be performed. Additionally, researchers are now interested in "lab-on-chip" detection model that would allow on-site analysis without the use of costly instrumentation and complicated protocols. Devising an appropriate technique would allow qualitative as well as quantitative estimation of analytes.

ACKNOWLEDGMENTS

The author acknowledges the remarkable work in the domain of nanosensing that had led to numerous research publications which have been highlighted in this chapter. The author would also like to thank DST-SERB, Govt. of India for fellowship under National Postdoctoral (NPDF) Scheme.

REFERENCES

Agrawal, Shailaja, Paknikar Kishore and Bodas Dhananjay, 2014. "Development of immunosensor using magnetic nanoparticles and circular microchannels in PDMS." *Microelectronics Engineering*. 115: 66–69. doi: 10.1016/j.mee.2013.10.020.

Ai, Kelong, Liu, Yanlan and Lu, Lehui, 2011. "Hydrogen-Bonding Recognition-Induced Color Change of Gold Nanoparticles for Visual Detection of Melamine in Raw Milk and Infant Formula." *J. Am. Chem. Soc.* 131: 9496–9497. doi: 10.1021/ja9037017

Akbarzadeh, Abolfazl, Samiei, Mohamad, and Daravan, Soodabeh, 2012 "Magnetic nanoparticles: preparation, physical properties, and applications in biomedicine." *Nanoscale Res. Lett.* 7: 1–13. doi: 10.1186/1556-276X-7-144.

Alivisatos, A. Paul. Johnsson, P. Kai, Peng, Xiagang. Wilson, E. Troy, Loweth, J. Colin., Bruchez, P. Marcel, Schultz, G. Peter. 1996. "Organization of 'nanocrystal molecules' using DNA." *Nature* 382: 609–611. doi: 10.1038/382609a0

Ambashta, D. Ritu and Sillanpaa, Mika. 2010. "Water purification using magnetic assistance: a review." Journals of Hazardous Materials 180: 38-49. doi: 10.1016/j.jhazmat.2010.04.105.

Azzazy, M. E. Hassan, and Mansour, M. H. Mai, 2009. "*In vitro* diagnostic prospects of nanoparticles." *Clin. Chim. Acta* 403: 1-8. doi: 10.1016/j.cca.2009.01.016.

Baptista, P. V., Doria, G., Quaresma, P., Cavadas, M., Neves, C. S., Gomes, I., Eaton, P., Pereira, E., and Franco, R. 2011. "Nanoparticles in molecular diagnostics." *Prog. Mol. Biol. Transl. Sci.*104: 427-488. doi:10.1016/B978-0-12-416020-0.00011-5.

Beveridge, S. Jacob, Stephens, R. Jason and Williams, E. Mary, 2011. "The use of magnetic nanoparticles in analytical chemistry." *Annual Review of Analytical chemistry* 4: 251–273. doi:10.1146/annurev-anchem-061010-114041.

Boisselier, E. and Astruc, D., 2009. "Gold nanoparticles in nanomedicine: Preparations, imaging, diagnostics, therapies and toxicity." *Chem. Soc. Rev.* 38: 1759-1782. doi: 10.1039/b806051g.

Bruchez, Marcel, Moronne, Mario, Gin, Peter, Weiss, Shimon and Alivisatos, Paul A., 1998. "Semiconductor Nanocrystals as Flurescent Biological Labels." *Science* 281: 2013–2016. doi: 10.1126/science.281.5385.2013.

Chauhan, Nidhi, Narang Jagriti and Pundir, C. S., 2011. "Immobilization of rat brain acetylcholinesterase on porous gold-nanoparticle – $CaCO_3$ hybrid material modified Au electrode for detection of organophosphorous insecticides." *Int. J. Biol. Macromol.* 49: 923 – 929. doi: 10.1016/j.ijbiomac.2011.08.006.

Chen, Hao, Xie, Yujie, Kirillov, M. Alexander, Liu Liangliang, Yu Minghui, Liu Weisheng and Tang, Yu, 2015. "A ratiometric fluorescent nanoprobe based on terbium functionalized carbon dots for highly sensitive detection of an anthrax biomarker." *Chem. Commun.* 51: 5036-5039. doi: 10.1039/C5CC00757G.

Chen, K. Chuan, Huang, Chih Ching and Chang, H. T., 2010. "Label-free colorimetric detection of picomolar thrombin in blood plasma using a gold nanoparticle-based assay." *Biosensors and Bioelectronics* 25:1922–1927. doi: 10.1016/j.bios.2010.01.005.

Cho, W. S., Cho, M. and Jeong J, et al., 2010. "Size-dependent tissue kinetics of PEG-coated gold nanoparticles" *Toxicol Appl Pharmacol* 245: 116-23. doi: 10.1016/j.taap.2010.02.013.

Choi, Jihye, Jaemoon Yang, Doyeon Bang, Joseph Park, Suh, Jinsuck Ssuck, Huh, Yongmin and Haam, Seungjoo, Haam 2012. "Targetable gold nanorods for epithelial cancer therapy guided by near-IR absorption imaging." *Small* 8:746–753. doi: 10.1002/smll.201101789.

Colombo, Miriam, Carregal-Romero, Susana, Casula, F. Maria, Gutierrez, Lucia, Morales, P. Maria, Bohm, B. Ingrid, Heverhagen, T. Johannes, Prosperi, Davide and Parak, J. Wolfgang. 2012. "Biological applications of magnetic nanoparticles." *Chemical Society Reviews* 12: 4306-4334. doi. 10.1039/c2cs15337h.

Conde, Joao, Rosa, Joao, Lima, C. Joao and Baptista, V. Pedro. 2012. "Nanophotonics for Molecular Diagnostics and Therapy Applications." *Int. J. Photoenergy*. 619530. doi:10.1155/2012/619530.

Dabbousi, O. B., Rodriguez-Viejo, J., Mikulec, F. V., Heine, J. R., et al., 1997. "(CdSe) ZnS Core−Shell Quantum Dots: Synthesis and Characterization of a Size Series of Highly Luminescent Nanocrystallites." *J. Phys. Chem. B* 101: 9463–9475. doi: 10.1021/jp9 71091y.

Dai, Hong, Yang, Caiping, Tong, Yuejin, Xu, Guifang, Ma, Xiuling, Lin Yanyu and Chen, Guonan., 2012. "Label-free electrochemiluminescent immunosensor for α-fetoprotein: performance of Nafion–carbon nanodots nanocomposite films as antibody carriers." *Chem. Commun.* 48: 3055-3057. doi: 10.1039/C1CC16571B.

Dai, Qiu, Liu, Xiong, Coutts, Janelle, Austin, Lauren and Huo, Qun, 2008. "A One-Step Highly Sensitive Method for DNA Detection Using Dynamic Light Scattering."*J. Am. Chem. Soc.*130: 8138–8139. doi: 10.1021/ja801947e.

Dasary S. R. Samuel, Singh K. Anant, Senapati Dulal, Yu Hongtao and Ray C. Paresh. 2009. "Gold nanoparticle based label-free SERS probe for ultrasensitive and selective detection of trinitrotoluene. " *J. Am. Chem. Soc.* 131:13806 – 13812. doi: 10.1021/ja905134d.

Derfus, A. M., Chan, W. C. W. and Bhatia, S. N. 2004. "Probing the Cytotoxicity of Semiconductor Nanoparticles." *NanoLett.* 4, 11-18. doi: 10.1021/nl0347334.

Dong, Yongqiang, Ruixue, Wang, Geli, Li, Congqiang, Chen, Yuwu Chi and Guonan Chen., et al., 2012. "Polyamine-functionalized carbon quantum dots as fluorescent probes for selective and sensitive detection of copper ions." *Anal. Chem.* 84: 6220 -6224. DOI:10.1021/ ac3012126.

Du, A. Bao, Li, Zheng Ping and Liu, Cheng Hui., 2006. "One-step homogeneous detection of DNA hybridization with gold nanoparticle probes by using a linear light-scattering technique." *Angew. Chem. Int. Ed.* 45: 8022–8025. doi: 10.1002/anie.200603331.

Du, Dan, Chen Shizhen, Cai Jie and Zhang, Aidong, 2008a. "Electrochemical Pesticide Sensitivity Test Using Acetylcholinesterase Biosensor Based on Colloidal Gold Nanoparticle Modified Sol-Gel Interface," *Talanta* 74: 766-772. doi: 10.1016/j.talanta.2007.07.014.

Du, Dan, Chen Shizhen, Song Dandan, Li Haibing and Chen, Xi, 2008b. "Development of Acetylcholinesterase Biosensor Based on CdTe Quantum Dots/Gold Nanoparticles Modified Chitosan Microspheres Interface." *Biosensors and Bioelectronics* 24: 475-479. doi: 10.1016/ j.bios.2008.05.005.

Duarte, Katia, Justino, I. L. Celine, Freitas C. Ana, Durate, C. Armando, Rocha-Santos, A. P. Teresa, 2014. "Direct reading methods for analysis of volatile organic compounds and nanoparticles: a review." *Trends Anal. Chem.* 53: 21–32. doi: 10.1016/j.trac.2013.08.008.

Dubertret, Benoit, Skourides, Paris, Norris, J. David, Noireaux, Vincent, Brivanlou H. Ali and Libchaber Albert, 2002. "In vivo imaging of quantum dots encapsulated in Phospholipid micelles." *Science* 298:1759 – 1762. doi: 10.1126/science.1077194.

Elghanian, Robert, Storhoff, J. James, Mucic, C. Robert, Letsinger, L. Robert and Mirkin, A. Chad. 1997. "Selective Colorimetric Detection of Polynucleotides Based on the Distance-Dependent Optical Properties of Gold Nanoparticles." *Science* 277:1078-1081. doi:10. 1126/science.277.5329.1078.

Freeman, Ronit, Liu, Xiaoqing and Willner, Itamar, 2011. "Amplified multiplexed analysis of DNA by the exonuclease III-catalyzed regeneration of the target DNA in the presence of functionalized semiconductor quantum dots." *Nano Lett.*11: 4456–4461. doi. 10.1021/nl202761g.

Gao, Xiang, Ding, Changqin, Zhu, Anwei, Tian, Yang, 2014. "Carbon-dot-based ratiometric fluorescent probe for imaging and biosensing of superoxide anion in live cells." *Anal. Chem.* 86: 7071-7078. doi: 10.1021/ac501499y.

Goldman, R. Ellen, Medintz, L. Igor, Whitley, L. Jessica, Hayhurst, Andrew, Clapp. R. Aaron, Uyeda, Tetsuo H., Deschamps, R. Jeffrey, Lassman, E. Michael and Mattous, Hedi, 2005. "A Hybrid Quantum

Dot−Antibody Fragment Fluorescence Resonance Energy Transfer-Based TNT Sensor." *J. Am. Chem. Soc.* 127: 6744–6751. doi: 10.1021/ja043677l.

Gooding, J. Justin, Shein Jarred, Lai M. H. Leo, 2009. "Using nanoparticle aggregation to give an ultrasensitive amperometric metal ion sensor." *Electrochem. Commun.* 11:2015 – 2018. doi: 10.1016/j.elecom.2009.08.043.

Haiss, W., Thanh, T. K. N., Aveyard, J. and Fernig, D. G. 2007. "Determination of Size and Concentration of Gold Nanoparticles from UV−Vis Spectra." *Anal. Chem. 79*: 4215–4221. Doi: 10.1021/ac07 02084.

Ho, Yi-Ping and Leong, W. Kam, 2010. "Quantum dot-based theronostics." *Nanoscale* 2: 60 –68. doi: 10.1039/B9NR00178F.

Hosseini, M. S. and Kamali, M., 2015. "Synthesis and characterization of aspartic acid-capped CdS/ZnS quantum dots in reverse micelles and its application to Hg(II) determination." *Journal of Luminescence*, 167: 51-58. doi: 10.1016/j.jlumin.2015.06.009.

Huang, Chih-Ching and Chang, Huan-Tsung, 2007. "Parameters for selective colorimetric sensing of mercury (II) in aqueous solutions using mercaptopropionic acid-modified gold nanoparticles." *Chem. Commun.* 1215-1217. doi: 10.1039/B615383F.

Huang, Chih-Ching, Huang Yu-Fen, Cao, Zehui, Tan Weihong and Chang, Huan-Tsung, 2005. "Aptamer-modified gold nanoparticles for colorimetric determination of platelet-derived growth factors and their receptors." *Anal Chem* 77: 5735–5741. doi: 10.1021/ac050957q.

Huang, Qitong, Hu SHirong, Zhang Hanqiang, Chen Jianhua, He Yasan, Li Feiming, Weng, Wen, Ni Jiancong, Bao Xiuxiu and Lin Yi., 2013. "Carbon dots and chitosan composite film based biosensor for the sensitive and selective determination of dopamine."*Analyst* 138: 5417-5423. doi: 10.1039/C3AN00510K.

Issadore, David, Chung Jaehoon, Shao Huilin, Liong Monty, Ghazani A. Arezou, Castro M. Cesar, Weissleder, Ralph and Lee Hakho, 2012. "Ultrasensitive clinical enumeration of rare cells ex vivo using a μ-Hall detector." *Sci. Transl. Med.* 141: 1–22. doi: 10.1126/scitranslmed. 3003747.

Jain, K. K. 2007. "Applications of nanobiotechnology in clinical diagnostics." *Clin. Chem.* 53: 2002–2009. doi: 10.1373/clinchem. 2007.090795.

Jain, K. Kewal. 2008. "Nanomedicine: Application of nanobiotechnology in medical practice." *Med. Princ. Pract.* 17: 89–101. doi: 10.1159/000112961.

Jena, K. B. and Raj, R. C., 2006. "Electrochemical biosensor based on integrated assembly of dehydrogenase enzymes and gold nanoparticles." *Anal Chem* 78: 6332–6339. doi: 10.1021/ac052143f.

Justino, I. L. Celine, Rocha-Santos, A. P. Teresa, Cardoso, Susana, and Duarte, C. Armando, 2013. "Strategies for enhancing the analytical performance of nanomaterial-based sensors." *Trends Anal. Chem.* 47: 27–36. doi: 10.1016/j.trac.2013.02.004.

Kalluri, J. R., Arbneshi, T., Khan, S. A., Neely, A., Candice, P., Varisli, B., Washington, M., McAfee, S., et al., 2009. "Use of Gold Nanoparticles in a Simple Colorimetric and Ultrasensitive Dynamic Light Scattering Assay: Selective Detection of Arsenic in Groundwater." *Angew. Chem. Int. Ed.* 48:1–5. doi: 10.1002/anie.200903958.

Khomutov, G. B. and Gubin, S. P., 2002. "Interfacial synthesis of noble metal nanoparticles." *Materials Science and Engineering: C*, 22: 141-146. doi: 10.1016/S0928-4931(02)00162-5.

Kim, H. Joong and Chung H. Bong., 2011. "Naked eye detection of mutagenic DNA photodimers using gold nanoparticles." *Biosens. Bioelectron.* 26: 2805-2809. doi: 10.1016/j.bios.2010.11.019.

Kim, S. Yeon, Kim, H. Joong, Kim A. In, Lee J. Su, Jurng Jongsoo and Gu, 2010. "A novel colorimetric aptasensor using gold nanoparticle for a highly sensitive and specific detection of oxytetracycline." *Biosensors and Bioelectronics* 26:1644–1649. doi: 10.1016/j.bios. 2010.08.046.

Kim, Youngjin, Robert, C. and Hupp. T. Joseph., 2001. "Gold nanoparticle-based sensing of "spectroscopically silent" heavy metal ions." *Nano. Lett.* 1: 165 – 170. https://www.scholars.

northwestern.edu/en/publications/gold-nanoparticle-based-sensing-of-spectroscopically-silent-heavy.

Kuzyniak, Weronika, Adegoke, Oluwasesan, Sekhosana, Kutloana, D'Souza Sarah, Tshangana, C. Sesethu, Hoffmann Bjorn et al., 2014. "Synthesis and characterization of quantum dots designed for biomedical use." 466: 382-389. doi: 10.1016/j.ijpharm.2014.03.037.

Li, Fei-Ming, Liu, J., Wang, X., Lin, L., Cia, W., Lin, X., Zeng, Yi, Li, Z and Lin, S. 2011. "Non-aggregation based label free colorimetric sensor for the detection of Cr (VI) based on selective etching of gold nanorods." *Sensors and Actuators B: Chemical.* 155 (2): 817-822. doi: 10.1016/j.snb.2011.01.054.

Li, Haitao, He Xiaodie, Kang Zhenhui, Huang Hui, Liu Yang et al., 2010. "Water-Soluble Flurescent Carbon Quantum Dots and Photocatalyst Design." *Angew. Chem. Int. Ed.* 49: 4430. doi: 10.1002/anie.20090 6154.

Li, Haitao, Kang Zhenhui, Liu Yang and Lee Shuit-Tong., 2012. "Carbon nanodots: synthesis, properties and applications." *J. Mater. Chem.* 22: 24230. doi: 10.1039/C2JM34690G.

Li, Linbo, Wang Chao, Liu Kangyu, Wang, Yuhan, Liu Kun, Lin Yuqing, 2015. "Hexagonal cobalt oxyhydroxide−carbon dots hybridized surface: high sensitive fluorescence turn-on probe for monitoring of ascorbic acid in rat brain following brain ischemia." *Anal. Chem.* 87: 3404. doi: 10.1021/ac5046609.

Li, Xiao-Hua, Xie Zonghong, Min Hong, Li Chenxin, Liu Meichuan, Xian Yuezhong and Jin Litong, 2006. "Development of Quantum Dots Modified Acetylcholi nesterase Biosensor for the Detection of Trichlorfon." *Electroanalysis* 18: 2163-2167. doi: 10.1002/elan.200 603615.

Li, Xiao-Shui, Zhu Gang-Tian, Luo Yan-Bo, Yuan, Bi-Feng and Feng, Yu-Qi. 2013. "Synthesis and applications of functionalized magnetic materials in sample preparation." *Trend. Anal. Chem.* 45: 233–247. doi:10.1016/j.trac.2012.10.015.

Li, Yuanpeng, Srinivasan Balasubramanian, Jing Ying, Yao Xiaofeng, Hugger A. Marie, Wang Jian-Ping and Xing Chengguo, 2010.

"Nanomagnetic competition assay for low-abundance protein biomarker quantification in unprocessed human sera." *J. Am. Chem. Soc.* 132: 4388–4392. doi: 10.1021/ja910406a.

Li, Zi, Yu Huijin, Bian Tong, Zhao Yufei, Zhou Chao et al., 2015. "Highly luminescent nitrogen-doped carbon quantum dots as effective fluorescent probes for mercuric and iodide ions."*J. Mater. Chem. C*, 3: 1922-1928. doi: 10.1039/C4TC02756F.

Lim, Y. Shi, Shen, Wei and Gao, Zhiqiang, 2015. "Carbon quantum dots and their applications." *Chem. Soc. Rev.* 44: 362-381. doi: 10.103 9/C4CS00269E.

Lin, Yiyang, Chapman Robert and Stevens M. Molly, 2015. "Integrative Self-Assembly of Graphene Quantum Dots and Biopolymers into a Versatile Biosensing Toolkit." *Adv. Func. Mater.* 25: 3183- doi: 10.10 02/adfm.201500624.

Liu X. Ma, C., Yan, Y., Yao, G., Tang, Y., Huo, P., Shi, W., and Yan, Y. 2013. "Hydrothermal Synthesis of CdSe Quantum Dots and Their Photocatalytic Activity on Degradation of Cefalexin. " *Ind. Eng. Chem. Res.* 52: 15015–15023. doi: 10.1021/ie4028395.

Liu, C.; Cao, H.; Li, Y. P.; Zhang, Y. 2006. "Gold nanoparticles/multi-wall carbon nanotubes modified pyrolytic graphite electrode as an electrochemical sensor for nitrobenzene determination." *J. N. Mater. Electrochem. Syst.* 9: 139 – 144. doi: http://ir.ipe.ac.cn/handle/122 111/3986

Liu, Dingbin, Qu Weisi, Chen Wenwen, Zhang Wei, Wang Zhuo and Jiang, Xingyu, 2010. "Highly Sensitive, Colorimetric Detection of Mercury (II) in Aqueous Media by Quaternary Ammonium Group-Capped Gold Nanoparticles at Room Temperature."*Anal. Chem.* 82: 9606-9610. doi: 10.1021/ac1021503.

Liu, Guodong, Mao, Xun, Phillips, A. Joseph, Xu. Hui, Tan, Weihong and Zeng, Lingwen, 2009. "Aptamer-nanoparticle strip biosensor for sensitive detection of cancer cells." *Anal. Chem.* 81:10013–10018. doi: 10.1021/ac901889s.

Liu, Juewen and Lu Yi, 2003. "A colorimetric lead biosensor using DNAzyme-directed assembly of gold nanoparticles." *J. Am. Chem. Soc.* 125: 6642 – 6643. doi: 10.1021/ja034775u.

Liu, Juewen and Lu, Yi .2006b. "Fast colorimetric sensing of adenosine and cocaine based on a general sensor design involving aptamers and nanoparticles." *Angew Chem Int Ed* 45: 90–94. doi: 10.1002/anie.20 0502589.

Liz-Marzan, M. Luis., 2006. "Tailoring surface plasmons through the morphology and assembly of metal nanoparticles." *Langmuir* 22: 32-41. doi: 10.1021/la0513353.

Loweth, J. Colin., Caldwell, W. Brett., Peng, Xiaogang, Alivisatos, A. Paul. and Schultz, G. Peter., 1999. "DNA-Based Assembly of Gold Nanocrystals." *Angew. Chem., Int. Ed.* 38: 1808–1812. doi.org/10.1 002/(SICI)1521-3773(19990614)38:12<1808::AID-ANIE1808>3.0.C O;2-C.

Lu, Wenbo, Qin, Xiaoyun, Liu, Sen, Chang, Guohui, Zhang, Yingwei, Luo, Yonglan, Asiri, Abdullah M., Al-Youbi, Abdulrahman Obaid, Sun, Xuping 2012. "Economical, green synthesis of fluorescent carbon nanoparticles and their use as probes for sensitive and selective detection of mercury (II) ions." *Anal. Chem.* 84: 5351-5357. doi: 10.1021/ac3007939.

Mariotti, Elisa, Minunni Maria and Mascini, Marco, 2002. "Surface Plasmon resonance biosensor for genetically modified organism's detection." *Anal Chim Acta.* 453:165–172. doi: 10.1016/S0003-2670(01)01458-1.

Mauriz, E., Calle, A., Manclus, J. J, Montoya, A. and Lechuga, M. L. 2007. "Multi-analyte SPR immunoassays for environmental biosensing of pesticides." 387:1449-1458. doi: 10.1007/s00216-006-0800-z.

Medintz, L. Igor, Clapp, R. Aaron, Mattoussi, Hedi, Goldman, R. Ellen, Fisher, Brent and Mauro, J. Mattew, 2003. "Self-assembled nanoscale biosensors based on quantum dot FRET donors."*Nat. Mater* 2: 630–638. doi: 10.1038/nmat961.

Medintz, L. Igor, Clapp, R. Aaron, Mattoussi, Hedi, Goldman, R. Ellen, Fisher, Brent and Mauro, J. Matthew, 2003. "Self-assembled nanoscale biosensors based on quantum dot FRET donors." *Nat. Mater.*, 2003, 2: 630– 638. doi: 10.1038/nmat961.

Muzyka, Kateryna, 2014. "Current trends in the development of the electrochemioluminescent immunosensors." *Biosensors and Bioelctronics* 54: 393–407. doi: 10.1016/j.bios.2013.11.011.

Newman, Janelle, Roberts, J. M. and Blanchard, J. Gary, 2007. "Optical organophosphate sensor based upon gold nanoparticle functionalized fumed silica gel." *Analytical Chemistry* 79: 3448 – 3454. doi: 10.1021/ac062165h.

Oliveira, M. M., Ugarte, D., Zanchet, D. and Zarbin, J. G. A., 2005. "Influence of synthetic parameters on the size, structure, and stability of dodecanethiol-stabilized silver nanoparticles." *Journal of Colloid and Interface Science*, 292: 429-435. doi: 10.1016/j.jcis.2005.05.068.

Pan, Dengyu, Zhang Jingchun, Li Zhen, Wu Chao, Yan Xiumei and Wu Minghong, 2010. "Observation of pH-, solvent-, spin-, and excitation-dependent blue photoluminescence from carbonnanoparticles."*Chem. Commun.* 46: 3681-3683. doi: 10.1039/C000114G.

Perez, J. M., Josephson, L., O'Loughlin, T., Hogemann, D., and Weissleder, R., 2002 "Magnetic relaxation switches capable of sensing molecular interactions." *Nature Biotechnol.* 20: 816 –820. doi: 10.1002/cbic.200300730.

Prasuhn, E. Duane, Feltz Anne, Blanco-Canosa B. Juan, Susumu Kimihiro, Stewart H. Michael, Mei C. Bing et al., 2010"Quantum Dot Peptide Biosensors for Monitoring Caspase 3 Proteolysis and Calcium Ions."*ACS Nano* 4: 5487–5497. doi: 10.1021/nn1016132.

Priyadarshini, E., and Pradhan. N. 2016, Gold Nanoparticles as efficient sensors in colorimetric detection of toxic metal ions: A Review. *Sensors and Acutators B,* 238: 888-902. doi: 10.1016/j.snb. 2016.06.081.

Priyadarshini, Eepsita and Rawat Kamala, 2017. "Au@carbon dot nanoconjugates as dual mode enzyme-free sensing platform for Cholesterol."*J. Mater. Chem. B*5: 5425-5432. doi: 10.1039/ C7TB01345K.

Qian, Zhaosheng, Chai, Lujing, Tang Cong, Huang Yuanyuan, Chen, Jianrong and Feng, Hui et al., 2015. "Carbon quantum dots-based recyclable real-time fluorescence assay for alkaline phosphatase with adenosine triphosphate as substrate." *Anal. Chem.* 87: 2966-2973. doi: 10.1021/ac504519b.

Reddy H. L., Arias L. Jose, Nicolas, Julien, and Couvreur, Patrick, 2012. "Magnetic nanoparticles: design and characterization, toxicity and biocompatibility, pharmaceutical and biomedical applications." *Chem. Rev.* 112: 5818-5878. doi: 10.1021/cr300068p.

Regulacio, D. Michelle and Han, Ming-Yong, 2010. "Composition-Tunable Alloyed Semiconductor Nanocrystals." *Acc. Chem. Res.,* 43: 621–630. doi: 10.1021/ar900242r.

Rocha-Santos, T. A. P., 2014. "Sensors and biosensors based on magnetic nanoparticles." *TrAC Trends in Analytical Chemistry*, 62: 28-36. doi: 10.1016/j.trac.2014.06.016.

Ronkainen, N. J., Halsall, H. B. and Heineman, R. W., 2010. "Electrochemical biosensors." *Chemical Society Reviews* 39:1747-1763. doi: 10.1039/B714449K.

Schmid, G. 1994. Clusters and colloids -From theory to applications. VCH Verlagsgesellschaft, Weinheim. (Schimd 1994 232).

Schmid, Gunter, and Lehnert, D. C. Andreas, 1989. "The Complexation of Gold Colloids." *Angew. Chem., Int. Ed.* 28: 609–611. doi: 10.1002/anie.198907801.

Shankaran, R. Dhesingh and Miura, Norio. 2007. "Trends in interfacial design for surface plasmon resonance based immunoassay." J. Phys. D: *Appl. Phys*. 40: 7187-7200. doi: JPhysD/40/7187.

Shao, Xiangling, Gu Hui, Wang Zhen, Chai Xiaolan, Tian Yang, Shi Guoyue, 2013. "Highly selective electrochemical strategy for monitoring of cerebral Cu^{2+} based on a carbon dot-TPEA hybridized surface." *Anal. Chem.* 85: 418-425. doi: 10.1021/ac303113n.

Shawky, M. Sherif, Bald Dirk, Azzazy, M. E. Hassan, 2010. "Direct detection of unamplified hepatitis C virus RNA using unmodified gold nanoparticles." *Clin. Biochem.* 43: 1163-1168. doi: 10.1016/j.clinbiochem.2010.07.001.

Shi, Wenbing, Wang, Qinlong, Long, Yijuan, Cheng, Zhiliang, Chen, SHihong, ZHeng, Huzhi and Huang, Yuming. 2011 "Carbon nanodots as peroxidase mimetics and their applications to glucose detection."Chemical Communications 47: 6695-6697. doi: 10.1039/C1 CC11943E.

Shyh-Dar, L. and Huang, L. 2011. "Stealth Nanoparticles: High Density but Sheddable PEG is a Key for Tumor Targeting" *J Control Release*. 145: 178–181. doi:10.1016/j.jconrel.2010.03.016.

Storhoff, J. J., Lucas, A. D., Garimella, V., Bao, Y. P. and Muller, U. R., 2004 "Homogeneous detection of unamplified genomic DNA sequences based on colorimetric scatter of gold nanoparticle probes." *Nature Biotechnol* 22*:* 883–887 doi. 10.1038/nbt977.

Sun, Jiefang, Guo, Lei, Bao, Yi and Xie, Jianwei, 2011. "A simple, label-free AuNPs-based colorimetric ultrasensitive detection of nerve agents and highly toxic organophosphate pesticide." *Biosensors and Bioelectronics* 28: 152–157. doi: 10.1016/j.bios.2011.07.012

Sun, Xiangying, Liu, Bin and Xia, Kaihao, 2011. "A Sensitive and Regenerable Biosensor for Organophosphate Pesticide Based on Self Assembled Multilayer Film with CdTe as Fluorescence Probe." *Luminescence* 26: 616-621. doi: 10.1002/bio.1284.

Sun, Xiaolian, Ho Don, Lacroix Lise-Marie, Xiao Q. John and Sun Shouheng, 2012. "Magnetic nanoparticles for magnetoresistance-based biodetection." *IEEE Trans. Nanobiosci.* 11: 46–53. doi: 10.1109/ TNB.2011.2176509.

Sun, Yugang and Xia, Younan, 2002. "Shape-Controlled Synthesis of Gold and Silver Nanoparticles." *Science* 298: 2176–2179.

Templeton, C. Allen, Wuelfing P. W., Murray W. Royce, 2000. "Monolayer-Protected Cluster Molecules." *Acc. Chem. Res.* 33: 27–36. doi: 10.1021/ar9602664.

Tholouli, E., Sweeney, E., Barrow, E., Clay, V., Hoyland, J. A., and Byers, R. J., 2008. "Quantum dots light up pathology." *Journal of Pathology*. 216:275–285. doi: 10.1002/path.2421.

Turkevich, John, Garton, G., Stevenson, C. Peter, 1954. "The color of colloidal gold." *J. Colloid Sci.* 9: 26-35. doi:10.1016/0095-8522 (54)90070-7.

Valera, Enrique, Ramon-Azcon, Javier, Sanchez, F. J. Marco, M. P. and Rodriguez Angel, 2008. "Conductimetric Immunosensor for Atrazine Detection Based on Antibodies Labelled with Gold Nanoparticles," *Sensors and Actuators B* 134: 95-103. doi: 10.1016/j.snb.2008.04.023.

Wang, Guang-Li., Dong, Yu-Ming, Zhu, Xiao-Ying, Zhang, Wen-Jing, Wang Cheng and Jiao, Huan-Jun., 2011. "Ultrasensitive and selective colorimetric detection of thiourea using silver nanoprobes." *Analyst* 136: 5256-5260. doi: 10.1039/C1AN15613F.

Wang, Y, Hu, R, Lin, G, Roy, I and Yong, K, 2013. "Functionalized Quantum Dots for Biosensing and Bioimaging and Concerns on Toxicity." *ACS Appl. Mater. Interfaces* 5: 2786–2799. doi:10.1021/am 302030a.

Wang, Youfu and Hu Aiguo, 2014. "Carbon quantum dots: synthesis, properties and applications." *J. Mater. Chem. C* 2: 6921 – 6939. doi: 10.1039/C4TC00988F.

Wei, Fang, Lam, Robert, Cheng, Stacy, Lu, Steven, Ho. Dean and Li, Na., 2010. "Rapid detection of melamine in whole milk mediated by unmodified gold nanoparticles." *Appl. Phys. Lett.* 96: 133702, doi:10. 1063/1.3373325.

Wilcoxon, Jess. 2009. "Optical absorption properties of dispersed gold and silver alloy nanoparticles." *J. Phys. Chem. B* 113: 2647-2656. doi: 10.1021/jp806930t.

Wu, W., Wu, Z., Yu, T., Jiang, C., and Kim, W. 2015. "Recent progress on magnetic iron oxide nanoparticles: synthesis, surface functional strategies and biomedical applications." *Sci. Technol. Adv. Mater.* 16: 023501. doi: 10.1088/1468-6996/16/2/023501.

Wu, Yuangen, Zhan, Shenshan, Wang Faze, He Lan, Zhi, Wenting and Zhou, Pei. 2012. "Cationic polymers and aptamers mediated aggregation of gold nanoparticles for the colorimetric detection of arsenic (III) in aqueous solution." *Chem. Commun.* 48: 4459–4461. doi: 10.1039/C2CC30384A.

Xia, Fan, Zuo Xiaolei, Yang Renqiang, Xiao Yi, Kang Di, Vallee-Belisle Alexis, Gong Xiong et al., 2010. "Colorimetric detection of DNA, small molecules, proteins, and ions using unmodified gold nanoparticles and conjugated polyelectrolytes." *Proc. Natl. Acad. Sci.* 107, 10837-10841. doi: 10.1073/pnas.1005632107.

Xiao, Lehui., Wei, Lin., He, Yan., and Yeung, S. Edward., 2010. "Single Molecule Biosensing Using Color Coded Plasmon Resonant Metal Nanoparticles." *Anal. Chem. 82:* 6308–6314. doi: 10.1021/ac101018v.

Xu, Quan, Pu, Peng, Zhao, Jungang, Dong Chenbo, Gao, Chun, Chen Yusheng, Chen, Jiarui, Liu Yao and Zhou, Hongjun., 2015. "Preparation of highly photoluminescent sulfur-doped carbon dots for Fe (III) detection." *J. Mater. Chem. A* 3:542-546. doi: 10.1039/C 4TA05483K.

Xu, Yuanhong, and Wang Erkang, 2012. "Electrochemical biosensors based on magnetic micro/nano particles." *Electrochim. Acta.* 84: 62–73. doi: 10.1016/j.electacta.2012.03.147.

Yu, Chengju and Tseng, Weilung, 2008. "Colorimetric Detection of Mercury (II) in a High-Salinity Solution Using Gold Nanoparticles Capped with 3-Mercaptopropionate Acid and Adenosine Monophosphate." *Langmuir* 24:12717-12722. doi: 10.1021/la802105b.

Yu, K. Mi, Kim, Dongkyun, Lee In-Hyun, So Jee-Soo, Jeong Y. Yong and Jon Sangyong, 2011. "Image-guided prostate cancer therapy using aptamer-functionalized thermally cross-linked superparamagnetic iron oxide nanoparticles."*Small* 7: 2241–2249. doi.org/10.1002/smll.20110 0472.

Yu, L., Ren, G., Tang, M., Zhu, B., Chai, F., Li Gang and Xu, D. 2018 "Effective Determination of Zn^{2+}, Mn^{2+}, and Cu^{2+} Simultaneously By Using Dual-Emissive Carbon Dots as Colorimetric Fluorescent Probe." *European Journal of Inorganic Chemistry*. doi: 10.1002/ejic.20180 0474.

Zamfir, Lucian-Gabriel, Geana Irina, Bourigua Sondes, Rotariu Lucian, Bala Camelia, Errachid Abdelhamid and Jaffrezic-Renault, Nicole, 2011. "Highly sensitive label-free immunosensor for ochratoxin A based on functionalized magnetic nanoparticles and EIS/SPR detection." *Sensors and Acutators B: Chemical* 159:178–184. doi:10.1016/j.snb.2011.06.069.

Zhang, Chun-yang and Johnson, W. Lawrence, 2009. "Single Quantum-Dot-Based Aptameric Nanosensor for Cocaine." *Anal. Chem.* 81: 3051– 3055. doi: 10.1021/ac802737b.

Zhang, Chun-Yang, Yeh, Hsin-Chih, Kuroki T. Marcos and Wang, Tza-Huei, 2005b "Single-quantum-dot-based DNA nanosensor." *Nat. Mater* 4: 826–831. doi: 10.1038/nmat1508.

Zhang, Haijuan, Chen, Yonglei, Liang, Meijuan, Xu, Laifang, Qi, Shengda, Chen, Hongli and Chen, Xingguo, 2014. "Solid-phase synthesis of highly fluorescent nitrogen-doped carbon dots for sensitive and selective probing ferric ions in living cells." *Anal. Chem.* 86: 9846. doi: 10.1021/ac502446m.

Zhang, Suxia, Wang Nu, Yu Huijun, Niu Yaming and Sun, Changqing, 2005a. "Covalent attachment of glucose oxidase to an Au electrode modified with gold nanoparticles for use as glucose biosensor." *Bioelectrochemistry* 67:15–22. doi: 10.1016/j.bioelechem.2004.12.002

Zhao, Weian, Karp, M. Jeffrey, Ferrari, Mauro, Serda, R.2011. "Bioengineering nanotechnology: Towards the clinic." Nanotechnology 22: 490201. doi: 10.1088/0957-4484/22/49/490201.

Zheng, Huzhi, Wang Qinlong, Long Yijuan, Zhang Haijie, Huang Xiaoxiao and Zhu Rui, et al., 2011. "Enhancing the luminescence of carbon dots with a reduction pathway." *Chem. Commun.* 47: 10650-10652. doi: 10.1039/C1CC14741B.

Zhong, X. H., Han, M. Y., Dong, Z., White, T. J., Knoll, W., 2003. "Composition-tunable Zn(x)Cd(1-x)Se nanocrystals with high luminescence and stability." *Journal of American Chemical Society.* 125: 8589- 8594. doi: 10.1021/ja035096m.

Zhou, Hankun, Gan ning, Li Tianhua, Cao Yuting, Zeng Saolin, Zheng Lei and Guo Zhiyong, 2012. "The sandwich-type electroluminescence immunosensor for a-fetoprotein based on enrichment by Fe3O4-Au magnetic nano probes and signal amplification by CdS-Au composite nanoparticles labeled anti-AFP." *Anal. Chim. Acta* 746: 107–113. doi: 10.1016/j.aca.2012.08.036.

Zhu, Anwei, Qu, Qiang, Shao Xiangling, Kong Biao and Tian Yang., 2012. "Carbon Dot Based Dual-Emission Nanohybrid Produces a Ratiometric FLurescent Sensor for In Vivo Imaging of Cellular Copper Ions." *Angew. Chem. Int. Ed.* 51: 7185-7189. doi: 10.1002/anie.201109089.

Zrazhevskiy, Pavel, Sena Mark and Gao Xiaohu, 2010 "Designing multifunctional quantum dots for bioimaging, detection, and drug delivery."*Chem. Soc. Rev.* 39: 4326–4354. doi:10.1039/B915139G.

In: Nanoparticles ISBN: 978-1-53616-596-8
Editors: A. K. Samantara, S. Ratha

Chapter 2

NANOPARTICLES AND THEIR APPLICATIONS IN THERAPEUTICS

Animesha Rath[1,*], Ipsita Mohanty[1] and Manas Ranjan Prusty[2]

[1]Regional Medical Research Centre (ICMR), Bhubaneswar, India
[2]Institute of Plant Science, Agricultural Research Organisation, Volcani, Israel

ABSTRACT

Nanoparticles are sub-microscopic particles made up of biocompatible materials like silica, metal, or crystals of 1–100 nm dimension range. Large surface area to mass ratio, exceptionally small size, and high reactivity are some of the exclusive properties of nanoparticles that have helped overcome the limitations of diagnostic agents used in traditional methods. The use of nanoscale sized particles has enabled us to modify the basic properties of materials such as diffusivity, solubility, and immunogenicity. The selectivity and specificity of nanoparticles towards a particular target has imparted the nanoparticles with anticancer effects besides reducing therapeutic

* Corresponding Author's Email: rath.animesha685@gmail.com.

toxicity. Precise engineering of materials at nanoscale, otherwise known as nanotechnology, has led to the development of novel therapeutic and diagnostic modalities producing medicines termed as "nanomedicine." The advantageous application of nanoparticles *viz.* enhancing the specificity by conjugating with the targeting ligands, improved stability and halflives after being coated with polymers, ability to be loaded with therapeutics, low polydispersity, potential to overcome drug resistance, and well-defined characterization methodologies help reduce health care costs. The last two decades have witnessed the treatment of number of health complications like diabetes, cancer, asthma, allergy, pain, infections, and many more through nanoparticle-based therapeutic and diagnostic agents. Nanoparticles have found applications in diagnostic approaches by helping identify anomalies such as precancerous cells, disease markers and fragments of viruses that cannot be detected by traditional diagnostics. Ever since the development of the nanoparticles, a number of therapeutic based products have been introduced to the pharmaceutical market, and numerous other products are still under clinical trials. Currently, nanotechnologies have found application in molecular diagnostic methods, such as DNA and protein microarray biochips. This chapter is focused on recent advances and novel nanoparticle therapeutics in use, clinical trial, or preclinical stage for disease and diagnostic applications.

Keywords: therapeutic, nanomedicine, treatment, diagnosis, cancer

1. Introduction

Nanotechnology is best defined with the understanding and control of matter at dimensions usually in the range of 1–1000 nm. Due to characteristic properties that are peculiar, and the ability to be loaded with therapeutics (coated with polymers to improve stability and half-lives) for diseases, nanoparticles have established itself in wide range of applications. Besides these nanoparticles also exhibit the properties of being conjugated to targeting ligands to enhance specificity, established characterization methodologies and low polydispersity, The application of nanotechnology to synthesize medicines at sub-micrometer length scale is concerned with the development of novel therapeutic and diagnostic modalities (Farokhzad and Langer 2006, 1456; Liu 2007, 2527). With the development and engineering of novel as well as unique therapeutic and diagnostic agents, these Nano medicines can overcome the challenges encountered by the traditional modalities. These therapeutic methods make use of nanomaterials to target the delivery of drugs more precisely in order to improve their solubility, half-life, therapeutic index, and to reduce their immunogenicity (Davis 2008, 771; Zhang 2008, 761; Park 2009, 410; Wang 2009, 3165). Ultra small size, large surface area to mass ratio, and high reactivity are some of the unique physicochemical properties of nanomaterials, which can be used to overcome several limitations of traditional therapeutic and diagnostic agents.

The last two decades have experienced the development of numerous nanoparticle-based therapeutic and diagnostic agents for the treatment of cancer, diabetes, pain asthma, allergy, infections, etc. (Davis 2008, 771; Brannon-Peppas and Blanchette 2004, 1649). In therapeutics, nanoparticles are delivered in a controlled manner to the targeted organ. Unlike traditional diagnosis, the approach made with these nanoparticles works out even at a molecular range, *viz.* identifying fragments of viruses, precancerous cells, and disease markers. The first generation nanoparticles, used for the diagnosis, are primarily based on liposomes and polymer–drug conjugates. Liposomes are spherical vesicles with a lipid bilayer membrane that can encapsulate both hydrophilic and hydrophobic agents, protecting the cargo (i.e., drugs comprising minute molecules, nucleotides, proteins, imaging agents or radio nucleotides) during their circulation in the body (Kawasaki and Player 2005, 101; Zhang 2008; 761). They target specific cells and tissues after being attached with ligands that direct themto the particular cell surface receptors. Additionally, they can be coated with polymers enhancing the circulation half-life. Liposome-encapsulated doxorubicin (Doxil; Ortho Biotech) had been approved by the US Food and Drug Administration (FDA) in 1995 for the treatment of HIV-related Kaposi's sarcoma, and was subsequently approved for the treatment of ovarian cancer and multiple myeloma. The extensive investigation on polymer-drug conjugates helped received regulatory approval (Kawasaki and Player 2005, 101; Torchilin 2005, 145; Duncan 2006, 688; Lammers and Ulbrich 2010, 119; Kopecek and Kopeckova 2010, 122).

Table 1. List of nanoparticles-based therapeutics approved by the FDA

Composition	Trade name	Company	Indication	Administration
Liposomal platforms				
Liposomal amphotreicin B	Abelcet	Enzon	Fungal infections	i.v.
	AmBisome	Gilead Sciences	Fungal and protozola infections	i.v.
Liposomal cytaratine	DepoCyt	Skye Pharma	Malignant lymphomatous meningitis	i.t.
Liposomal daunorunicin	DounoXome	Gilead Sciences	HIV-related Kaposi's sarcoma	i.v.
Liposomal doxorubicin	Myocet	Zeneus	Combination therapy with cyclophosphemide in metastatic breast cancer	i.v.
Liposomal IRIV vaccine	Epaxal	Berna Biotech	Hepatis A	i.m.
	Inflexal V	Berna Biotech	Influenza	i.m.
Liposomal morphine	DepoDur	Skye Pharma, Endo	Post-surgical analgesis	Epidural
Liposomal vertepofin	Visudyne	QLT, Novartis	Age related macular degeneration, pathologic myopia, ocular histoplasmosis	i.v.
Liposome-PEG doxorubicin	Doxil,Caelyx	Ortho Biotech, Schering-Plough	HIV-related Kaposi's sarcoma, metastatic breast cancer, metastatis ovarian cancer	i.m.
Micellular estradiol	Estrasorb	Novavax	Menopausal therapy	Topical
Polymeric patforms				
L-Glutamic acid, L-alanine, L-Lysine, and L-tyrosine copolymer	Copaxone	TEVA Pharmaceuticals	Multiple sclerosis	s.c.

Composition	Trade name	Company	Indication	Administration
Methoxy-PEG-poly(o,L-lactide) taxol	Genexol-PM	Samyang	Metastatic breast cancer	i.v.
PEG-adenosine deaminase	Adagen	Enzon	Severe combined immunodeficiency disease associated with ADA deficiency	i.m.
PEG-anti-VEGF aptamer	Macugen	OSI Pharmaceuticals	Age related macular degeneration	i.t.
PEG-a-interferon 2a	Pegasys	Nektar, Hoffmann-La Roche	Hepatitis B, hepatitis C	s.c.
PEG-GCSF	Neulasta	Amgen	Neutropenis associated with cancer chemotherapy	s.c.
PEG-HGF	Somavert	Nektar,Pfizer	Acromegaly	s.c.
PEG-L-asparaginase	Oncaspar	Enzon	Acute lymphoblastic leukemia	i.v.,i.m.
Poly(allylamine hydrochloride)	Renagal	Genzyme	End-stage renal disease	Oral
Other platforms				
Albumin-bound paclitaxel	Abraxane	Abraxis BioScience,AstraZeneca	Metastatic breast cancer	i.v
Nanocrystalline aprepitant	Emend	Elan,Merck	Antiernetic	Oral
Nanocrystalline fenofibrate	Tricor	Elan, Abbott	Anti-hyperlipidemic	Oral
Nonocrystalline sinolimus	Rapamune	Elan, Wyeth Pharmaceuticals	Immunosuppressant	Oral

Growth factor, HIV, human immunodeficiency virus, i.m., intramuscular, i.v., intravenous, IRIV, immunopotentiating reconstituted influenza virosome, i.t., intrathecal, PEG, polyethylenegylcol, s.c., subcutaneous, VEGF, vascular endothelial growth factor.

The most widely studied polymer for this application is polyethylene glycol (PEG), which can enhance the solubility and plasma stability of proteins, and reduce immunogenicity. PEG-1 asparaginase (Oncospar; Enzon) is the first nanoparticle therapeutic to have FDA approval in 1994, for the treatment of acute lymphocytic leukaemia (Duncan 2006, 688; Kopecek and Kopeckova 2010, 122). Liposomes and polymer–drug conjugates have provided the base for advanced drug delivery by encapsulation of cargo coupled with activated release. However, with the development of next generation nanoparticles therapeutics, based on polymeric nanoparticles that combine the pre-eminent features of traditional delivery vectors, offer improved flexibility to overcome some of the key barriers in the field. A progressive increase in the number of commercially available nanoparticle-based therapeutic products has been seen in the past two decades. Liposomal drugs and polymer–drug conjugates account for more than 80% of the total amount of available products (Table 1).

2. Classification of Nanoparticles

On the basis of composition nanoparticles are classified into several categories, i.e., carbon based, metal based, dendrimers and composites.

2.1. Carbon Based Nanoparticles

Composed mostly of carbon, these nanomaterials are commonly found in the form of hollow spheres, ellipsoids, or tubes (Bhaviripudi 2007, 1516). These are mainly classified into fullerenes, graphene, carbon nano tubes (CNT), carbon nanofibers, carbon black, and sometimes, nano-sized activated carbon (Figure 1). Cylindrical carbon nanomaterials are categorized as nanotubes, whereas spherical and ellipsoidal carbon nanomaterials are referred to as fullerenes. These carbon based nanoparticles have found to be effective in many fields of interest, e.g., electronics, improvised films and coatings and stronger and lighter materials.

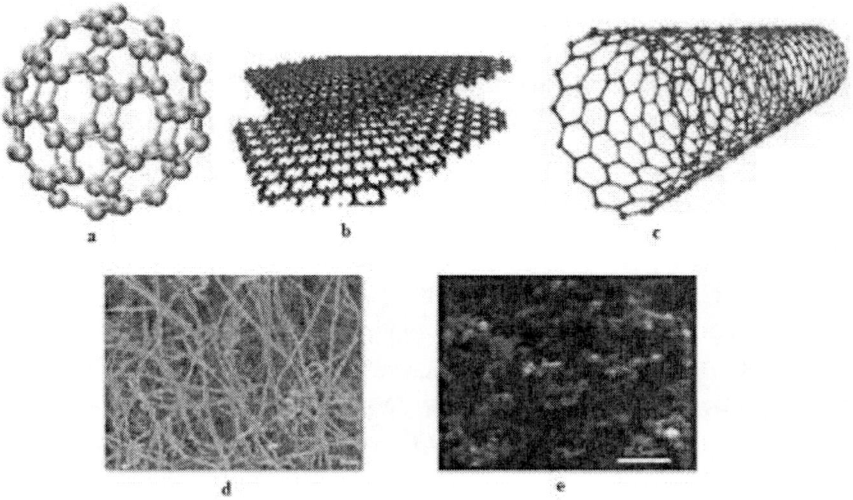

Figure 1. Carbon based nanoparticles (a) fullerenes (b) graphene (c) carbon nanotubes (d) carbon nanofibers and (e) carbon black.

2.1.1. Fullerenes

Fullerenes (C_{60}) consist of carbon atoms held together by sp^2 hybridization and are spherical in shape. Anti-human immunodeficiency virus (HIV) activity is one of most potential aspects exhibited by C_{60}. C_{60} derivatives, which are water soluble, inhibit HIV protease activity by binding to its active site owing to their unique molecular structure and hydrophobicity (Schinazi 1993, 1707). Fullerenes target HIV enzymes like reverse transcriptase is known to have anti-HIV activity (Jensen 1996, 767). Due to conformational complementarity and size similarity, fulleres binds to the active site of HIV-1 protease thus inhibiting viral protease.

2.1.2. Graphene

Graphene, an allotrope of carbon, is a network of honeycomb lattice made up of carbon atoms in a two dimensional surface. Due to its robust yet flexible physico-chemical properties, graphene has been extensively used for engineering thin and flexible materials (Kim 2009, 706; Eda 2008, 270). Oxidation of graphite under acidic conditions leads to the production of graphene oxide (GO) that offers several advantages over using pure graphene (Dreyer 2010, 228). The hydrophilic functional groups and structural heterogeneity of graphene oxide facilitates chemical functionalization and imparts broad range of physical properties. Graphene has also been widely used in several types of sensors and biosensors (e.g., optical, chemical, and piezoelectric).

2.1.3. Carbon Nano Tubes

Chemical vapor deposition of graphite or arc discharge could yield carbon nanotubes. Arc discharge between graphite electrodes together using an yttria-nickel catalyst synthesizes carbon nanotubes under an Ar-H_2 gases mixture atmosphere that is created using different pressure and DC currents. A graphene nano foil/sheet is wrapped/rolled up to produce hollow cylinders, called carbon nanotubes having diameters, 0.7 nm (for a single layered CNT), and 100 nm (for multi-layered CNT) with length varying from a few micrometers to several millimeters. The ends of the synthesized tubes can either be closed by a half fullerene molecule or remain hollow. CNTs have many industrial applications due to their broad range of physical and chemical properties (Baughman 2002, 787). High-efficiency electron emission devices such as electron microscopes, flat display panels, and gas-discharge tubes are comprised of CNTs. Carbon nanotubes are also used in light emitting elements/devices as they display strong luminescence from field emission (Endo 2008, 13).

2.1.4. Carbon Nanofiber (CNFs)

The graphene nanofoils wound into a cone or cup shape are used to produce carbon nanofibers. The electrical properties of CNFs and their composites are mostly determined by their sensitivity (Wangxi 2003, 2805; Vilaplana 2013, 4776; Baeza 2013, 841; Endo 2001, 1287; Du 2002, 1232; Wu 2004, 81). Carbon nanofiber composites are used worldwide these days as electrode materials for batteries and supercapacitors. CNFs have also been applied as promising materials in many fields, such as reinforcement of composites, energy conversion and storage, self-sensing devices, sensors, electrode materials and electromagnetic shielding.

2.1.5. Carbon Black

These are small, spherical carbon based particles with diameters ranging from 20 to 70 nm and are primarily of amorphous nature. Strong interaction among these particles leads to the formation of agglomerates with a diameter of 500 nm. Several toxicity tests are carried out by implementing carbon black as an important reference material (i.e., Printex 90) (Nikula 1995, 80; Heinrich 1995, 80).

2.2. Metal and Metal Oxides Based Nanoparticles

Metal based nanoparticles are synthesized either by destructive and constructive methods from metals to nanometric sizes. In destructive method, bulk material which is decomposed into decreasingly smaller fragments by mechanical influences resulting objects of 100 nm diameter whilst in constructive method the nanoparticles are synthesized from simpler molecules where the shape and size of the nanoparticles can be controlled by varying the chemical composition and reaction conditions. Nanoparticles can be synthesized from almost all metals (Salavati-niasari 2008, 3514). Some of the common metals for nanoparticle synthesis are gold (Au), silver (Ag), aluminium (Al), iron (Fe), cadmium (Cd), copper (Cu), cobalt (Co), lead (Pb), and zinc (Zn). The nanoparticles synthesized from metals have distinctive properties such as high surface area to volume ratio, surface charge and surface charge density, crystalline and amorphous structures, reactivity, pore size, shapes, colour, etc. These nanoparticles also exhibit sensitivity to environmental factors such as air, sizes as low as 10 to 100 nm, moisture, heat and sunlight. The properties of metal based nanoparticles can be modified with the synthesis of metal oxide based nanoparticles. Increased reactivity and efficiency (Tai 2007, 5536) are the major advantages of metal oxide nanoparticles. For instance, reactivity of iron nanoparticles is significantly enhanced when iron (Fe) oxidises to form iron oxide (Fe_2O_3) in the presence of oxygen at room temperature. These nanoparticles possess exceptional properties when compared to their metal counterparts. The surface functionalization ability of these metallic nanoparticles enables their application in other related fields such as bioassays, detection, imaging and so on. The metal based nanoparticles are emerging as good carriers for drug delivery, and an integral part of the biosensor composites. Many metal-based nanoparticles have also been extensively studied for their application as novel antimicrobial (i.e., antiviral, antibacterial, antifouling, and antifungal) agents (Cioffi 2005, 5255; Anyaogu 2008, 4340; Alt 2004, 4383; Morones 2005, 2346; Son 2004, 1632). Some of the commonly synthesised metal based nanoparticles are aluminium oxide (Al_2O_3), cerium oxide (CeO_2), iron oxide (Fe_2O_3), magnetite (Fe_3O_4), silicon dioxide (SiO_2), titanium oxide (TiO_2), and zinc oxide (ZnO).

2.3. Dendrimers

The well-defined architecture and unique characteristics of Dendrimer leads to its emergence as another novel class of drug delivery nanoparticle platform (Kukowska-Latallo 2005, 5317; Bhadra 2006, 623; Dutta 2007, 89; Morgan 2006, 11913). In dendrimers, the chemical polymers are compartmentalized with multiple layers of repeating units, termed generation, having an active terminal group and an initiator core (denoted as generation zero). These are tree-like, hyper branched structures whose size and shape can be precisely controlled (Figure 2). The electrostatic adsorption or covalent conjugation of the multivalent surfaces of dendrimers facilitates to the process of carrying specific drugs to the target sites. Alternatively, the cavities in their cores can be loaded with drugs through hydrophobic interaction, hydrogen bond, or chemical linkage. Dendrimers cover various other distinct applications viz., solubilization, gene therapy, and immunoassay and MRI contrast agent.

Table 2. List of selected metal nanoparticles and their applications

Nanoparticle	Abbreviation	Application
Aluminium	Al	Fuel additive/Propellant, explosive, wear resistant coating additive
Gold	Au	Cellular imaging, Photodynamic therapy
Iron (oxide)	Fe, Fe_3O_4, Fe_2O_3	Magnetic imaging, environmental remediation
Silica	SiO_2	Fabrication of electric and thermal insulators, catyst supports, drug carriers, gene delivery, adsorbents, molecular sieves and filler materials
Silver	Ag	Anti microbial, photography, batteries, electrical
Copper	Cu	Antimicrobial (i.e., antiviral antibacterial, antifouling, antifungal), antibiotive treatment alternatives, nanocomposite coating, catalyst, lubricants, inks, filler materials for enhanced conductivity and wear resistance
Cerium (oxide)	CeO_2	Polishing and computer chip manufacturing, fuel additive to decrease emission
Manganese (oxide)	Mn	Catalysts, Batteries
Nickel (oxide)	Ni	Conduction, magnetic properties, catalysts, battery manufacturing, printing inks
Titanium dioxide	TiO_2	Photocatalyst, anti bacterial coating, sterilization, paint, cosmetics, sunscreens
Zinc (oxide)	Zn, ZnO	Skin protectant, sunscreen

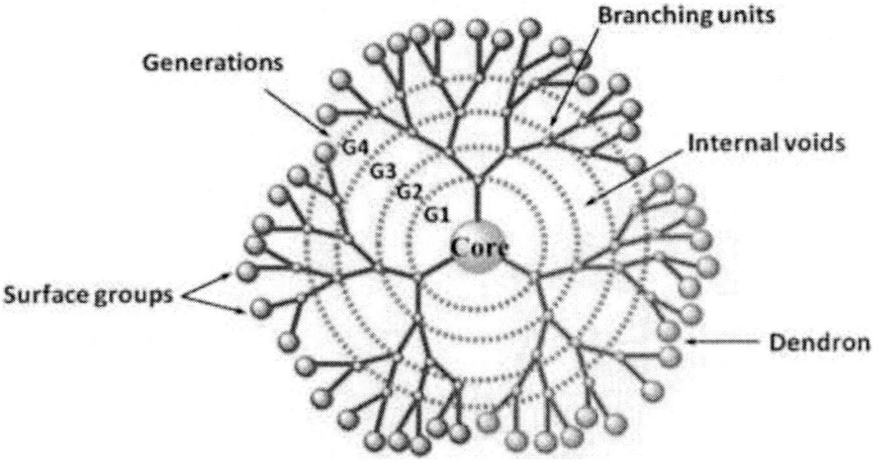

Figure 2. General architecture of a dendrimer (Adopted from Jain 2014, 2476).

2.4. Composites

Composite nanoparticles contain two or more nanoscale components having special physico-chemical properties. The structural features of these nanoparticles categorize them in the following groups: simple hybrid, core/shell structured composite nanoparticles, and multifunctional quantum dots (Figure 3). The dimension of some composite nanoparticles has been reduced to less than 1–20 nm, and has become much more complex referred to as quantum dots. The complexity of quantum dots arise from factors that includes chemical composition, oxidative, mechanical and photolytic stability, capping ligands, charge, size and concentration. The pivotal factors in determining the properties and functionalities of composite nanoparticles are composition, atomic order of the aggregates, and size. The nanoscale regime of composite nanoparticles confers structural and electronic degrees of freedom which are inaccessible to bulk materials. The mechanical, thermal, and flame retardant properties can be enhanced with an addition of nanosized clays to result products ranging from auto parts to packaging materials. With the development of microfluidic technologies, the synthesis of sub-micrometer-sized nanocomposites has become much affordable now-a-days.

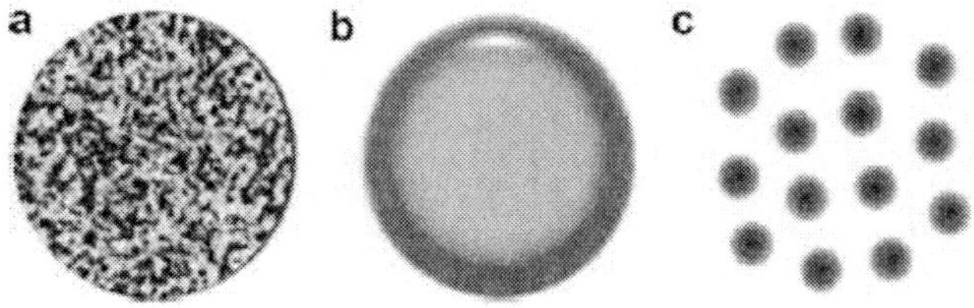

Figure 3. Composite nanoparticles (a) simple hybrid (10–100 nm); (b) core/shell structured (10–100 nm); (c) multifunctional quantum dots (1–20 nm).

3. Synthesis of Nanoparticles

The nanoparticles can be synthesized by following either of the Bottom-up or Top-down synthetic approaches (Figure 4). They are categorized mainly on the basis of the starting precursor chosen.

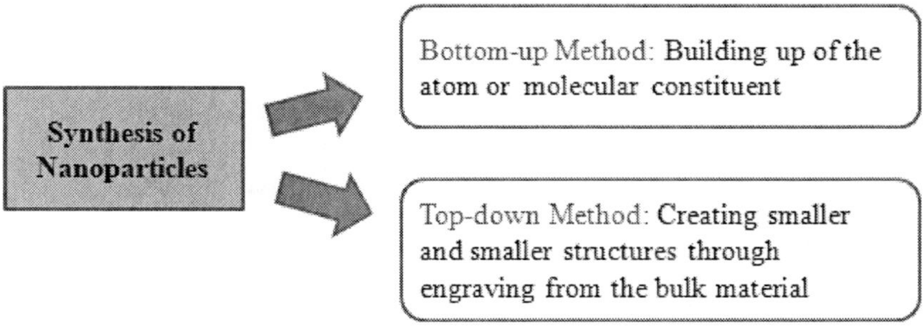

Figure 4. Methods for synthesis of nanoparticles.

3.1. Bottom-Up Synthesis Methods

3.1.1. Chemical Vapour Deposition

Chemical vapour deposition (CVD) is defined as a thermally induced chemical reaction that occurs at the surface of a heated substrate in the presence of gaseous reactants resulting in the formation of thin film. Thus a thin film of the required material could be afforded by this reaction, which is later recovered and used. The key influencing factor in CVD is the substrate temperature. The general steps involved in the CVD process and schematic diagram of a conventional CVD unit is presented in the following figure (Figure 5). The advantages of CVD are clearly visible from the uniform, strong, hard and highly pure nanoparticles it produces, while the requirement of special equipment and toxic and/or hazardous gaseous by-products are some of its major disadvantages (Adachi 2003, 77). This process is mostly used in the semiconductor industry for depositing thin films of various materials.

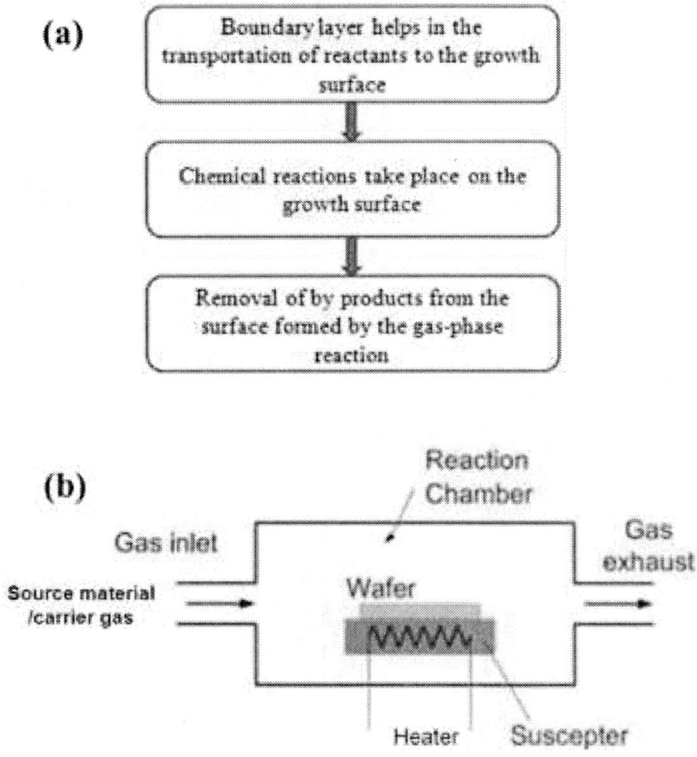

Figure 5. (a) Steps involved in CVD process and (b) Schematic diagram of a conventional CVD reactor. (Adopted from https://slideplayer.com/slide/4217130).

3.1.2. Sol-Gel Method

Sol-gel method is a chemical procedure that leads to the conversion of a solution to a gel like diphasic system containing both liquid and solid phase. In this method, the gel like properties can be recognized at initial phase after the removal of a significant amount of fluid from the solution. Being a low temperature technique, this method is cheap. The chemical composition of the product can be controlled in sol-gel method. Colloids appear bulky upon mixing with a liquid, whereas nanosized molecules, in most of the cases, form a clear (or near transparent) mixture. It leads to the evolution of networks through the formation of colloidal suspension (sol) and gelatin to form a network in continuous liquid phase (gel). The initial phase of the sol-gel process involves the preparation of a homogeneous solution of one or more selected alkoxides. The ions of metal alkoxides and aloxysilanes (tetramethoxysilane (TMOS), and tetraethoxysilanes (TEOS)) are the precursors for synthesizing these colloids. These alkoxides are organo-metallic precursors for silica, aluminum, titanium, zirconium, etc., and are immiscible in water (Bhargava 1994, 416; Yu 2001, 1890; Lu and Jagannathan 2002, 3608; Morita 2004, 5). A catalyst is used to trigger the reaction process and control the pH, while alcohol is used as a mutual solvent.

3.1.3. Pyrolysis

The large scale production of nanoparticles in industries relies mostly on pyrolytic techniques. In this process, the precursor can be either liquid or vapour, and is fed into the furnace at high pressure through a small hole where it is incinerated (Figure 6) (Kammler 2001, 583). Nanoparticles are recovered after the combustion or after air classification of by-product gases. For easy evaporation, some of the furnaces use plasma and laser instead of flame to produce high temperature (Amato 2013, 461). The advantages of pyrolysis are high-efficiency, cost effectiveness, simple, and continuous process with high yield.

3.1.4. Biosynthesis

This involves a green and environmental friendly approach where biodegradable and non-toxic nanoparticles are synthesized (Kuppusamy 2014, 473). Instead of conventional chemicals, unconventional resources such as bacteria, plant extracts, fungi, etc. are used as precursors to produce nanoparticle for bio-reduction and capping purposes. The nanoparticles produced through biosynthesis have unique and enhanced properties, making them suitable for biomedical applications (Hasan 2015, 9).

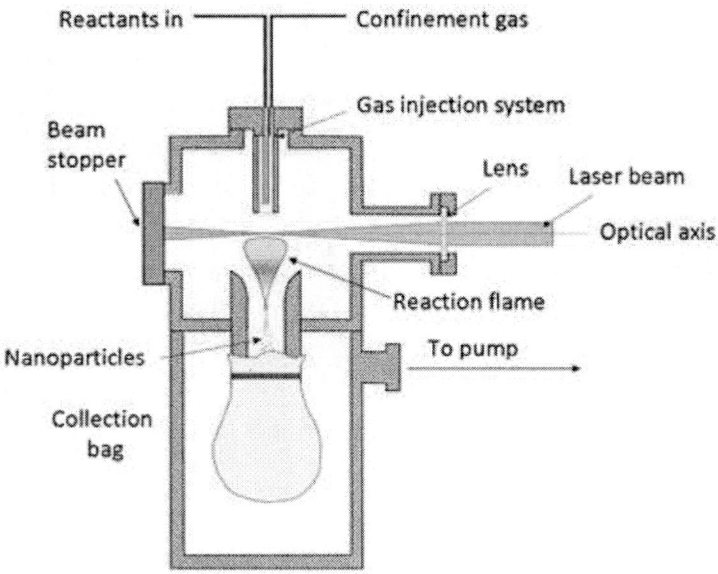

Figure 6. Synthesis of nanoparticles by pyrolysis (Adopted from Borsella 2011, 54. Open Access).

3.2. Top-Down Synthesis Methods

3.2.1. Mechanical Milling

One of the extensively used methods for making nanoparticles in the top down synthesis involves mechanical alloying/milling. This unique process is carried out at room temperature. During synthesis, an inert atmosphere is needed where different elements are milled, and mechanical milling is carried out for milling and annealing of nanoparticles (Yadav 2012, 22). In mechanical milling, nanostructures are produced as a result of plastic deformation by the structural decomposition of coarser grained structures instead of cluster assembly. The mechanical alloying processes, i.e., rod milling and ball milling techniques have received much attention as a powerful tool for the fabrication of several advanced materials. The influencing factors in mechanical milling include fracture that leads to decrease in particle size, cold-welding leading to increase in particle size and plastic deformation that leads to particle shape.

3.2.2. Thermal Decomposition

Thermal decomposition is a heat driven endothermic chemical decomposition process, breaking the chemical bonds in the compound (Salavati-niasari 2008, 3514). The chemical decomposition of the element occurs at a specific temperature called decomposition temperature. Decomposing the metal at specific temperatures through suitable chemical reactions leads to the production of nanoparticles along with some secondary products.

3.2.3. Sputtering

Sputtering involves the ejection of ultra-small particles that are subsequently deposited on the surface of a target substrate under high vacuum conditions (Shah and Gayrin 2006, 118). In this process, a thin layer of nanoparticles is deposited on the surface of the substrate, and then annealed at desired temperature (Figure 7). The shape and size of the nanoparticles are determined by the thickness of the layer deposited, duration of annealing, substrate type, temperature, etc. (Lugscheider 1998, 398).

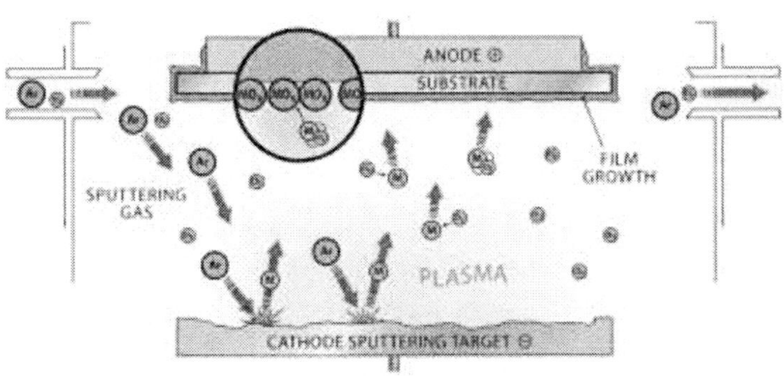

Figure 7. Schematic presentation showing the Sputtered deposition unit (Adopted from http://lnf-wiki.eecs.umich.edu/wiki/Sputter_deposition. Open Access).

4. Approaches of Nanoparticles Targeting

Functionalizing the nanoparticles with targeting ligands is one of the major strategies to improvise the therapeutic index of the yielded nanoparticles. Improving the efficacies of the available therapeutic agents and development of new diagnostic tools are the key focuses of nanoparticle synthesis. Addition of targeting ligands ensures the delivery of drug-encapsulated nanoparticles to uniquely identified sites with minimal undesired effects. Targeted drug delivery approaches are classified into three major categories; (i) mechanical or physical approach requiring a device for particulate delivery (ii) chemical approach which depends on enzymatic activation of ligands for targeting active biological molecules at specific target sites or organs using chemical delivery systems; (iii) biological approach which involve a carrier system like antibodies or lecithin for the delivery of the drug (Chandra 1991, 137). Approaches for targeting nanoparticles can be broadly classified into two areas; active and passive targeting (Figure 8).

4.1. Active Targeting

Identifying and interacting with a specific cell, tissue or organ in the body by employing active agents having selective affinity is referred to as active targeting. Import of thousands of drug molecules is facilitated by receptor targeted ligands that employs coupling of drug carrier nanosystems to ligands. Several moieties like vitamins, carbohydrates, aptamers, peptides (e.g., Arg-Gly-Asp, allatostatin, and transactivating transcriptional activator) and proteins (e.g., lectins, and transferrin) have been examined as targeting agents (Zhang 2007, 1889; Eliaz and Szoka 2001, 2592; Farokhzad 2006, 1456; Hu 2008, 797; Lu 2009, 87; Singh 2009, 645; Wang 2010, 11306; Ulbrich 2009, 251). However, active agents such as antibodies for surface proteins and ligands for the receptors have been used extensively to target specific cells. Active targeting can be accomplished in several ways. Recognizing the nature of cell surface receptors for which the drug will be targeted, enables active targeting of the affected tissue (Galvin 2011, 389). Cell-specific ligands can then be utilized for specific binding of nanoparticle to the cell having complementary receptor. Active targeting can also be achieved by utilizing magnetoliposomes, which serve as contrast agent in magnetic resonance imaging, where drug can be delivered to a region of the body with the help of magnetic positioning (Galvin 2011, 389).

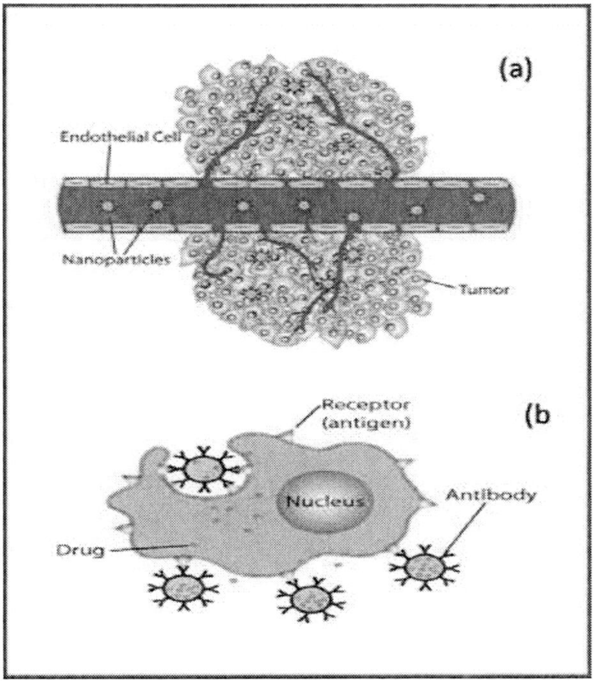

Figure 8. Passive targeting: nanoparticles directed towards the target tissue as a result of ineffective lymphatic drainage and vessel leakage, (b) Active targeting: nanoparticles targeting with conjugated antibodies (Adopted from Barakat 2012, 9).

4.2. Passive Targeting

Accumulation of drug or drug-carrier system at a particular site due to pharmacological or physico-chemical factors is referred to as passive targeting (Garnette 2001, 171; Kim 2008, 41). In passive targeting, ligand–

receptor interactions can be highly selective for precise targeting at the site of interest (Kaparissides 2006, 1). Multiple obstacles are encountered by the treated nanoparticles on their way to the target sites in passive targeting. These barriers include non-specific uptake of the particle, non-specific drug delivery due to uncontrolled release and mucosal barriers. Therefore, functionalization with antibodies and maintaining appropriate size can help in reducing non-specific toxicity and to provide an enhanced mode of drug delivery. In addition, the drug encapsulation must be done to ensure that the particle must not diffuse until it binds itself to the target. There are several advantages of drug targeting that include simplified drug administration protocol, low dose drug administration for efficient therapeutic effect, cost effectiveness and lessened side effects due to targeted drug delivery (Vasir 2005, 47).

5. Applications of Nanoparticles in Therapeutics

With nanotechnology, nanoparticles have emerged as attractive tools for providing solutions in pharmaceutics and biomedicines (Figure 9 and 10). The formulation of nanoparticles for drugs, proteins and hormone delivery make use of various polymers. Biodegradable synthetic polymers, such as poly(lactide-glycolide) (PLGA) copolymers, polyacrylates and poly(caprolactone)s (PCLs), or natural polymers, such as albumin, gelatin, alginate, collagen and chitosan offer targeted delivery to specific sites besides providing physical protection from environmental stimuli.

5.1. Cellular Targeting

5.1.1. Nanoencapsulation for Drug Delivery

With nano encapsulation, there is an increase in drug efficacy, specificity, therapeutic index and tolerability of corresponding drugs (Vijaykumar 2012, 111). Various patents for such nanoencapsulated drugs exist (Chungunpituk 2007, 139). Being nanocapsulated, these drugs are well protected from the interacting biological environment, and thus avoiding any premature degradation. Nanocapulation of drugs also improves intracellular penetration along with controlled delivery, bioavailability, and enhanced absorption into a selected tissue as well as the retention time (Safra 2000, 1029; Schroeder 1998, 1305; Raghuvanshi 2002, 109; Kreutera 1997, 81; Fasas 2003, 161; Leroux 1996, 339; Alexis 2008, 505). Nanomedicines for cancer, AIDS, malaria, diabetes, prion disease and tuberculosis are under trail phase with some of them being commercialized. Various polymeric nanoparticles (PLA, PLGA, PCA, chitosan, gelatin) with different drugs impart surface modification, bioavailability, and drug release mechanism. A higher encapsulation efficiency of 75% has been reported in the case of insulin loaded nanoparticles of PLGA, where PLGA has a functional role in maintaining the integrity of insulin during formulation and delivery (Podaralla 2006, 613). Mittal et al., 2007 (77) have reported Estradiol encapsulated PLGA nanoparticles that improves oral bioavailability and effectively reduces the frequency of the dose, while limiting dose dependent side effects and maximizing patient's compliance.

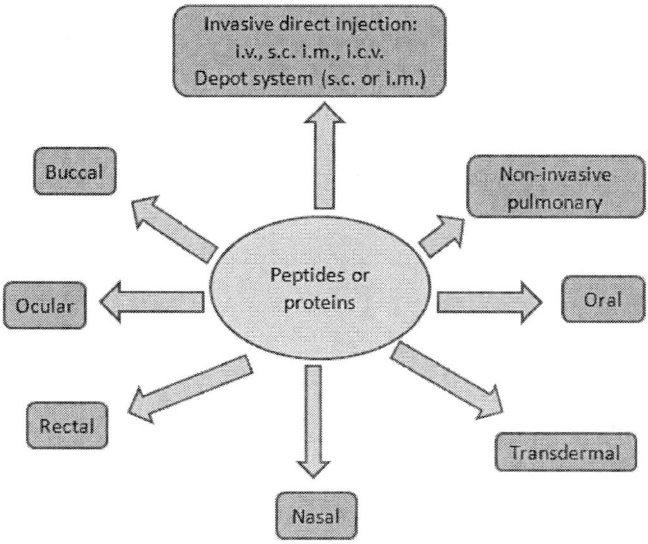

Figure 9. Delivery routes for therapeutic peptides and proteins (i.v.-intravenous, s.c.- subcutaneous, i.m.-intramuscular, i.c.v.- intra cerebral vein).

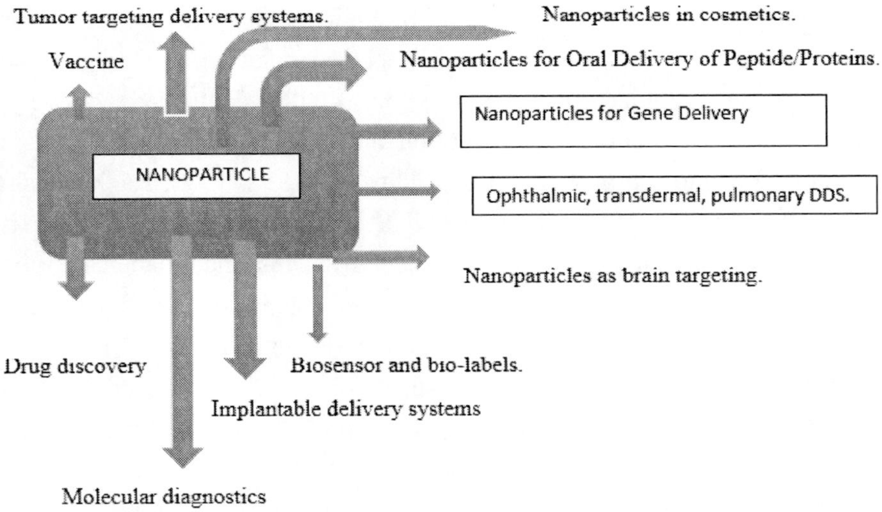

Figure 10. Application of nanoparticles in pharmaceutics (Adopted from Kumar 2015, 703) Open access.

5.1.2. Nanoparticles in Oral Delivery

Encapsulation of bioactive molecules with polymeric nanoparticles protects them against hydrolytic and enzymatic degradation by the gastrointestinal tract epithelial barriers. Damge et al., 1990 (233) have found that following an oral administration of insulin loaded nanoparticles; there has been a preservation of insulin activity and simultaneous reduction in the blood glucose level in diabetic rats for up to 14 days. Enhanced oral absorption and hypoglycemic activity of FA-PEG-PLGA-NPs encapsulated insulin (Folate coupled polyethylene glycolylated polylactide-coglycolide nanoparticles) exhibited a doubled oral bio-availability without any hypoglycemic shock. The gastrointestinal tract provides barrier for protein or peptide delivery viz., uptake of particulate matter from the environment is prevented by the M cells of small intestine. This gastrointestinal barrier can be overcome through nanoparticles that enhance the interaction mechanism of drug delivery system and the epithelial cells of the gastrointestinal tract.

5.1.3. Nanoparticles in Brain Delivery

The blood brain barrier is selectively permeable to small sized and lipophilic molecules from the blood circulated to the central nervous system (CNS), and is impermeable to water soluble drugs. PEG coated nanoparticles have been reported to deliver drugs to the brain. It slows down kidney ultrafiltration and enlargement of molecules allowing accumulation into the brain and other permeable tissues. It reduces proteolysis within the serum and tissues thus providing protein shielding and obstructs surface epitopes immune surveillance (Bhatt 2013, 2305).

5.1.4. Nanoparticles in Opthalmics

Nanoparticles play a vital role in overcoming poor solubility of drugs in lachrymal tissues. Nanoparticles offer a prolonged resident time in cul-de-sac for an effective treatment with respect to maintenance of the tonicity of the eye. The constant inflow and outflow of lachrymal fluids affects the intrinsic dissolution rate of the drug. Pignatello et al., 2006 (7) have stabilized chloricromene in ophthalmic formulations with an enhanced bioavailability by solvent evaporation method at ocular level. Eudragit RS 100 loaded piroxicam nanoparticles prepared by Adibkia et al., 2007 (407) helped in controlling the inflammatory symptoms in rabbits with endotoxin-induced-uveitis. Ophthalmologic formulation has a disadvantage of fast removal from the eye, clearing the applied drug through the nose. Nanoparticles' adhesiveness leads to higher drug levels at desired site of action. Alhough nanoparticles are of limited toxicological acceptance, yet Cavalli et al., (2002, 241) showed that solid lipid nanoparticles have a prolonged retention time in the eye, which was confirmed by using radiolabeled formulations and γ- scintigraphy. The lipids metabolize easily and open new ways for ophthalmological drug delivery without hampering vision (Araujo 2009, 56).

5.1.5. Nanoparticles in Topical Formulations

Creams and water-free ointments can be incorporated with nanoparticles which in turn lead to an increased solubility/diffusion of the drug when applied topically. Micellar nanoparticles (a multi-phase nanoemulsion) in topical applications allow a higher concentration of drug to penetrate the stratum corneum and epidermis creating a depot of drugs. By this, it avoids hepatic first-pass effects and contact with gastrointestinal tract thus proving to be acceptable by the patients (Muller 1999, 175). High permeability, large surface area and strong scattering pattern of solid lipid nanoparticles are effective in curing acne, atopic eczema and psoriasis. The solid lipid nano-forrmulations can further be incorporated into certain drugs (viz Vitamin A) to reduce their side effects (Shim 2004, 477; Kohli 2004, 13; Yamaguchi 2005, 29). Estrasorb is the world's first nano-engineered topical dosage form for hormone replacement therapy, approved by US FDA (Wright, 1997). Nanoparticle and nanocarriers mediated drug delivery to skin may bring a new direction for the treatment of several skin disorders (Papakostas 2011, 533).

5.1.6. Nanoparticles in Cosmetics

The occlusive nature and ultraviolet ray shielding properties of solid lipid nanoparticles allows their use in cosmetics. The permeability of these nanoparticles through dead skin layers allows for skin hydration. Wising (2003, 6) found that the solid lipid nanoparticles are effective carriers for cosmetic creams that enhance skin hydration. The particulate matter of these nanoparticles (focusing on its refractive index, size of particles and thickness of formulations on skin) provides physical protection in form of sunscreens that reflect and/or scatter UV rays. The solid lipid nanoparticles are better in scattering UV lights than liquid emulsion droplets (Patel 2006, 323). Besides their use in sunscreen (Popov 2005, 1), nanoparticles are also used in the manufacturing of breast cream (Gelis 2003, 242), hair care shampoo and conditioner (Nohynek and Schaefer 2001, 285), make-up kit, moisturizers/anti-wrinkle creams (Stober 1968, 62), toothpaste, and fullerenes (known for anti-aging properties).

5.1.7. Nanoparticles for Pulmonary Delivery

Alveoli, the functional unit of lungs, have rich vasculature, high epithelial permeability and surface area, which facilitate rapid absorption of nanoparticles. Moreover, the release and transport of the drugs are controlled by the size of the nanoparticles that are suitable for absorption. Some of the common drugs for this route are antiallergens (cromolyn sodium), bronchodialators (salbutamol) and steroidal anti-inflammatory agents (betamethasone) (Li 2010, 1977). The particle size of solid liquid nanoparticle is too small and can be exhaled. So, they cannot be administered to the lungs. Therefore, the solid lipid nanoparticles need to be aerosolized, but agglomeration of those nanoparticles must be prevented. Vibrating mesh-based nebulizers (*e.g.,* Aerogen nebulizer) offer potential for high efficiency delivery of aerosolized medications. After localization of the aerosolised nanoparticles in the bronchial tube and alveoli, the drug can be released in a controlled manner from the lipid particles (Gaumet 2008, 1).

5.2. Gene Delivery

Delivery of gene can be augmented by coupling plasmid DNA with nanoparticles that help in escaping to the cytoplasmic compartment without being subjected to the endolysosomal compartment (Panyam 2002, 1217). This escape helps the release of DNA at a sustained rate and enhances gene expression. PLGA nanoparticles containing therapeutic genes such as bone morphogenic proteins are delivered through this strategy which helps in bone healing.

5.3. Cancer Nanotechnology

Magnetic nanoparticles are used to diagnose and treat cancer. Magnetic nanoparticles are controlled by an external magnetic field gradient. These field gradients help transport magnetic nanoparticles into human tissues and concentrate them within the target tissues, especially the tumor or cancer cells. Magnetic iron oxide and gold nanoparticles can also detect the spread of such cancerous growth throughout the body. Encased in a biocompatible material, these nanoparticles help detect even smaller sized cancer cells. These nanoparticles get attached to the tumor cells turning them into little magnets that are then attracted to the tip of the biopsy needle (Charles 1986, 153). MRIs can be used rather than biopsies to detect malignant lymph nodes confirming its spread. The active targeting by ligands, retention effect and enhanced permeability of the nanoparticles help deliver a concentrated dose of drug in the vicinity of the targeted tumors, thereby reducing the exposure of drugs to healthy tissues, which limits the drug distribution only to the target organ. There are studies showing that the in-vivo drug distribution pattern is greatly influenced by several properties of nanoparticles like biodegradation profile, hydrophobicity and type of the polymer along with the molecular weight of the associated drugs, technique of incorporation mode, its localization in the nano spheres and adsorption. The bio-distribution of nanoparticles mostly involves mononuclear phagocytic system (MPS) and phagocytosis/ endocytosis/process, which is rapid (within 1 hour to 3 hours). However, the exact underlying mechanism behind the process is not fully understood. Such propensity of MPS for phagocytosis/ endocytosis of nanoparticles provides an opportunity for efficient and effective delivery of therapeutic agents. The chemotherapeutic treatment of MPS rich organs/tissues, digestive tract hepatic metastasis, gynecological cancers, hepatocarcinoma, primitive tumors, bronchopulmonary tumors, small cell tumors, leukemia and myeloma is greatly benefitted by the bio-distribution pattern of nanoparticles (Zhang 2001, 75).

5.4. Advantages of Nanoparticles

- Appropriate for administration through different routes (oral, nasal, parenteral etc.) (Paul 2004, 1).
- Enables both passive and active drug targeting after parenteral administration through manipulation of particle size and surface characteristics of nanoparticles.
- High carrying capacity.

- Better delivery of drugs to various anatomic extremities of body such as blood brain barrier (Rawat 2006, 1790).
- Increased shelf-stability of drug.
- Ability of controlled and sustainable patterns of drug release: They control the release of the drugs during the transportation to the site of localization, altering organ distribution and subsequent clearance of the drug so as to achieve increase in drug therapeutic efficacy and reduction in side effects.
- Suitable for co- delivery of two or more drugs (combination therapy)
- Can incorporate both hydrophilic and hydrophobic drugs.
- Enhances the bioavailability and precise targeting of drugs.
- Facilitates imaging related studies.
- Reduces drug toxicity and provides more efficient drug distribution through targeted nano drug carriers.
- Site-specific targeting by attaching targeting ligands to surface of the particles or by using magnetic guidance.
- Facilitates the development of safer class of medicines (Gelperina 2005, 1487; Susa 2009, 399; Sajja 2009, 43).
- Helps overcome the resistance offered by the physiological barriers in the body, since particle size directs the efficient delivery of drug to various parts of the body.
- Improves aqueous solubility of poorly soluble drugs.

5.5. Disadvantages of Nanoparticles

- High manufacturing costs which makes the product costlier.
- The preparation process utilizes solvents that are toxic in nature.
- Can alleviate allergic and immune responses in the body.
- May create toxicity issues through extensive use of poly (vinyl alcohol) as stabilizer.

- Particle-particle aggregation due to small size and large surface area may hinder the process of physical handling. (Mainardes 2005, 363; De Jong and Borm 2008, 133; Varde and Park 2004, 35).

5.6. Challenges

- Poor solubility.
- Inadequate in-vitro stability (self-life).
- Shorter in-vivo stability (half-life).
- Probability of aggravated side effects.
- Targeted delivery requirement.
- Regulatory related issues.
- Lack of mass production processes (Muller and Keck 2014, 151).

6. Perspectives

The potential application of nanotechnology has a broad spectrum in disease prevention, diagnosis and treatment. To obtain real progress, the practical application of nanomedicine needs visionary power, creativity, basic fundamental approach and systematic development. Basically, nanomedicine mainly relies on;

- Chemical knowledge that enables proper conjugation of drug/contrast agent through required modifications to the nanovector surface;
- Brief understanding of disease pathophysiology and biology for efficient therapy and targeting;
- Awareness on physical properties of multilevel nanosystems to enable fine manipulation for the design of new drug delivery and nanoscale detection systems.

Conclusion

Nanoparticles are extensively used in diagnostics, drug delivery, drug discovery and many other applications related to medical research. They are being used to produce anti-graffiti wall coatings, transparent sunscreens, stain repellent fabrics, ceramic coatings for solar cells, crack-resistant paints, self-cleaning windows, and scratch proof eyeglasses. The delivery of drugs to the desired sites in the body is still in a growing stage Farokhzad and Langer 2009, 16). In spite of significant challenges, the last five decades have witnessed several efforts in the design and application of nanoparticles.

References

Adachi M, Tsukui S, Okuyama K. 2003. "Nanoparticle Synthesis by Ionizing Source Gas in Chemical Vapor Deposition" *Jpn J Appl Phys* 42: L77-79, doi:10.1143/JJAP.42.L77.

Adibkia K, Reza M, Shadbad S, Nakhodchi A, Javadzedeh A, Jalali M B, Barar J, Mohammadi G, Omidi Y. 2007. "Piroxicam nanoparticles for ocular delivery: physiochemical, characterization and implementation in endotoxin induced uveitis" *J Drug Target* 15: 407-416, doi: 10.1080/10611860701453125.

Alexis F, Pridgen E, Molnar L K, Farokhzad O C. 2008. "Factors affecting the clearance and biodistribution of polymeric nanoparticles." *Mol Pharm* 5: 505-515, doi: 10.1021/mp800051m.

Alt V, Bechert T, Steinrucke P, Wagener M, Seidel P, Dingeldein E, Domann E, Schnettler R. 2004. "An *in vitro* assessment of the antibacterial properties and cytotoxicity of nanoparticulate silver bone cement." *Biomaterials* 18: 4383-4391, doi: 10.1016/j.biomaterials.200 3.10.078.

Amato R D, Falconieri M, Gagliardi S, Popovici E, Serra E, Terranova G and Borsella E. 2013. "Synthesis of ceramic nanoparticles by laser pyrolysis: From research to applications." *J Anal Appl Pyrolysis* 104: 461-469, doi: 10.1016/j.jaap.2013.05.026.

Anyaogu K C, Fedorov A V, Neckers D C. 2008. "Synthesis, characterization, and antifouling potential of functionalized copper nanoparticles." *Langmuir* 24: 4340-4346, doi: 10.1021/la800102f.

Araujo J, Gonzalez E, Egea M A, Garcia M L, Souto E B. 2009. "Nanomedicines for ocular NSAIDs: safety on drug delivery." *Nanomedicine* 45: 56-64, doi: 10.1016/j.nano.2009.02.003.

Baeza F J, Galao O, Zornoza E, Garcés P. 2013. "Multifunctional cement composites strain and damage sensors applied on reinforced concrete (RC) structural elements." *Materials* 6: 841-855, doi: 10.3390/ma6030841.

Barakat N S, Taleb D A B, Al Salehi A S. 2012. "Target Nanoparticles: An Appealing Drug Delivery Platform." *J Nanomedic Nanotechnol* S4: 009, doi: 10.4172/2157-7439.S1.07.

Baughman R H, Zakhidov A A, de Heer W A. 2002. "Carbon Nanotubes–The Route toward Applications." *Science* 297: 787-792, doi: 10.1126/science.1060928.

Bhadra D, Bhadra S and Jain N K. 2006. "PEGylated peptide dendrimeric carriers for the delivery of antimalarial drug chloroquine phosphate." *Pharm Res* 23: 623-33, doi: 10.1007/s11095-005-9396-9.

Bhargava R N, Gallagher D, Hong X and Nurmikko A. 1994. "Optical properties of manganese-doped nanocrystals of ZnS." *Physical Review Letters* 72: 416-419, doi: 10.1103/PhysRevLett.72.416.

Bhatt N, Ganesh B, Preeti K. 2013. "Drug delivery in the brain using polymeric nanoparticles: A review" *Int J Pharm Life Sci* 2: 2305-2330, doi: 10.3329/ijpls.v2i3.15457.

Bhaviripudi S, Mile E, Iii SAS, Zare A T, Dresselhaus M S, Belcher A M and Kong J. 2007. CVD Synthesis of Single-Walled Carbon Nanotubes from Gold Nanoparticle Catalysts." *J Am Chem Soc* 129: 1516-1517, doi: 10.1021/ja0673332.

Borsella E, D'Amato R, Fabbri F, Falconieri M, Terranova G. 2011. "Synthesis of nanoparticles by laser pyrolysis: from research to applications, Energ." *Ambient Innov* 4: 54-64. https://pdfs.

semanticscholar.org/b8fb/6d783d26f04fe6926bd2dc0f8055c5c235ff.pdf.

Brannon-Peppas L, Blanchette J O. 2004. "Nanoparticle and targeted systems for cancer therapy." *Adv Drug Deliv Rev* 56: 1649-1659, doi : 10.1016/j.addr.2004.02.014.

Cavalli R, Gasco M R, Chetoni P, Burgalassi S, Saettone M F. 2002. "Solid lipid nanoparticles (SLN) as ocular delivery system for tobramycin." *Int J Pharm* 238: 241-245, doi: 10.1016/S0378-5173(02)00080-7.

Chandra S, Agrawal A K, Gupta C M. 1991. "Chloroquine delivery to erythrocytes in Plasmodium berghei-infected mice using antibody-bearing liposomes as drug vehicles." *J Biosci* 16: 137-144, doi: 10.1007/BF02703366.

Charles S W and Popplewell J. 1986. "Properties and applications of magnetic liquid" *Handbook of magnetic materials* 2: 153, doi: 10.1016/0160-9327(82)90070-9.

Cannavale A, Fiorito F, Manca M, Tortorici G, Cingolani R, and Gigli G. 2010. "Multifunctional bioinspired sol-gel coatings for architectural glasses." *Building and Environment* 45: 1233-1243.

Chungunpituk J. 2007. "Nanosuspension technology for drug delivery." *Walailak J Science and Technology* 4: 139-153, doi: 10.2004/wjst.v4i2.94.

Cioffi N, Torsi L, Ditaranto N, Tantillo G, Ghibelli L, Sabbatini L, Bleve-Zacheo T, D'Alessio M, Zambonin P G, Traversa E. 2005. "Copper nanoparticle/polymer composites with antifungal and bacteriostatic properties." *Chem Mater* 17: 5255-5262, doi: 10.1021/cm0505244.

Damge C, Michel C, Aprahamian M, Couvrier P, Devissaguet J P. 1990. "Nanocapsules as carrier for oral peptide delivery." *J Control Release* 13: 233-239, doi: 10.1016/0168-3659(90)90013-J.

Davis M E, Chen Z, Shin D M. 2008. "Nanoparticle therapeutics: an emerging treatment modality for cancer." *Nature Rev Drug Discov* 7: 771-782, doi: 10.1038/nrd2614.

De Jong W H and Borm P J. 2008. "Drug delivery and nanoparticles:applications and hazards." *Int J Nanomedicine* 3: 133-149, doi: 10.2147/ijn.s596.

Dreyer D R, Park S, Bielawski C W, Ruoff R S. 2010. "The Chemistry of Graphene Oxide." *Chem Soc Rev* 39: 228-240, doi: 10.1039/ B917103G.

Du J H, Sun C, Bai S, Su G, Ying Z, Cheng H M. 2002. "Microwave electromagnetic characteristics of a microcoiled carbon fibers/paraffin wax composite in Ku band." *J Mater Res* 17: 1232-1236, doi:10.1557/JMR.2002.0182.

Duncan R (2006). Polymer conjugates as anticancer nanomedicines. *Nature Rev Cancer* **6:** 688-701, doi: 10.1038/nrc1958.

Dutta, T, Agashe, H. B., Garg, M., Balakrishnan, P., Kabra, M., Jain, N. K. 2007. "Poly (propyleneimine) dendrimer based nanocontainers for targeting of efavirenz to human monocytes/macrophages *in vitro*." *J Drug Target* 15: 89-98, doi: 10.1080/10611860600965914.

Eda, G., Fanchini, G., Chhowalla, M. 2008. "Large-Area Ultrathin Films of Reduced Graphene Oxide as a Transparent and Flexible Electronic Material." *Nat Nanotechnol* 3: 270-274, doi: 10.1038/nnano.2008.83.

Eliaz, R. E., Szoka F C Jr. 2001. "Liposome-encapsulated doxorubicin targeted to CD44: a strategy to kill CD44-overexpressing tumor cells." *Cancer Res* 6: 2592-2601. http://cancerres.aacrjournals.org/content/ 61/6/2592.long.

Endo M, Kim Y A, Hayashi T, Nishimura K, Matusita T, Miyashita K, Dresselhaus M S. 2001. "Vapor-grown carbon fibers (VGCFs): Basic properties and their battery applications." *Carbon* 39: 1287-1297, doi: 10.1016/S0008-6223(00)00295-5.

Endo, M.; Strano, M S.; Ajayan, P M. 2008. "Potential Applications of Carbon Nanotubes." In: Jorio, A.; Dresselhaus, G.; Dresselhaus, MS., editors. *Carbon Nanotubes: Advanced Topics in the Synthesis, Structure, Properties and Applications*. Springer; Berlin p. 13-61, doi: 10.1007/978-3-540-72865-8_2.

Farokhzad O C and Langer R. 2006. "Nanomedicine: developing smarter therapeutic and diagnostic modalities." *Adv Drug Deliv Rev* 58: 1456-1459, doi: 10.1016/j.addr.2006.09.011.

Farokhzad O C and Langer R. 2009. "Impact of nanotechnology on drug delivery." *ACS Nano* 3: 16-20, doi: 10.1021/nn900002m.

Farokhzad O C, Cheng J, Teply B A, Sherifi I, Jon S, Kantoff P W, Richie J P, Langer R. 2006. "Targeted nanoparticle-aptamer bioconjugates for cancer chemotherapy *in vivo*." *Proc Natl Acad Sci USA* 103: 6315-6320, doi: 10.1073/pnas.0601755103.

Fasas A, Buffels R, Kaloyannidis P, Anagnostopoulos A. 2003. "Safety of high dose liposomal Daunorubicin (Daunoxome) for refractory or relapsed acute myeloblastic leukemia for refractory or relapsed acute myeloblastic leukemia" *Br J Hematol* 122: 161-163, doi: 10.1046/ j.1365-2141.2003.04395_3.x.

Galvin P, Thompson D, Ryan K B, Mccarthy A, Moore A C, Burke C S, Dyson M, Maccraith B D, Gun'Ko Y. K, Byrne M T, Volkov Y, Keely C, Keehan E, Howe M, Duffy C, Macloughlin R. 2011. "Nanoparticle-Based Drug Delivery: Case Studies for Cancer and Cardiovascular Applications." *Cell Mol Life Sci* 69: 389-404, doi: 10.1007/s00018-011-0856-6.

Garnette M C. 2001. "Targeted drug conjugates: principles and progress." *Adv Drug Deliv Rev* 53: 171-216, doi: 10.1016/S0169-409X(01) 00227-7.

Gaumet M, Vargas A, Gurny R, Delie F. 2008. "Nanoparticles for drug delivery: the need for precision in reporting particle size parameters." *Eur J Pharm Biopharm* 69: 1–9, doi: 10.1016/j.ejpb.2007.08.001.

Gelis C, Girard S, Mavon A, Delverdier M, Paillous N, Vicendo P. 2003. "Assessment of photoprotective capacities of organo-mineral broadspectrum sunblock on two ex vivo skin models." *Photodermatol Photoimmunol Photomed* 19: 242-253, doi:10.1034/j.1600-0781.2003. 00045.x.

Gelperina S, Kisich K, Iseman M D, Heifets L. 2005. "The Potential Advantages of Nanoparticle Drug Delivery Systems in Chemotherapy of Tuberculosis." *Am J Respir Crit Care Med* 12: 1487-1490, doi: 10.1164/rccm.200504-613PP.

Hasan S. 2015. "A Review on Nanoparticles: Their Synthesis and Types." *Res J Recent Sci* 4: 9-11. http://www.isca.in/rjrs/archive/v4/iISC-2014/3.ISCA-ISC-2014-Poster-3BS-63.pdf.

Heinrich U, Fuhst R, Rittinghausen S, Creutzenberg O, Bellmann B, Koch W, Levsen K. 1995. *"Chronic inhalation exposure of Wistar rats and two different strains of mice to diesel engine exhaust, carbon black and titanium dioxide." Fundam Appl Toxicol* 25: 80-94, doi: 10.3109/08958379509015211.

Hu Z, Luo F, Pan Y, Hou C, Ren L, Chen J, Wang J, Zhang Y. 2008. "Arg-Gly-Asp (RGD) peptide conjugated poly(lactic acid)–poly(ethylene oxide) micelle for targeted drug delivery." *J Biomed Mater Res A* 85: 797-807, doi: 10.1002/jbm.a.31615.

Jain V and Bharatam P V. 2014. "Pharmacoinformatic approaches to understand complexation of dendrimeric nanoparticles with drugs." *Nanoscale* 6: 2476, doi: 10.1039/C3NR05400D.

Jana P, Aiman H, Müller R H. 2007. "Lipid nanoparticles (SLN, NLC) in cosmetic and pharmaceutical dermal products." *Int J Pharm* 366: 170-84, doi: 10.1016/j.ijpharm.2008.10.003.

Jensen A W, Wilson S R, Schuster D I. 1996. "Biological Applications of Fullerenes." *Bioorgan Med Chem* 4: 767-779, doi: 10.1016/0968-0896(96)00081-8.

Kammler B H K, Mädler L and Pratsinis S E. 2001. "Flame Synthesis of Nanoparticles." *Chem Eng Technol* 24: 583-596, doi: 10.1002/1521-4125(200106)24:6<583::AID-CEAT583>3.0.CO;2-H.

Kaparissides C, Alexandridou S, Kotti K, Chaitidou S. 2006. "Recent advances in novel drug delivery systems." *J Nanotechnol* 2: 1-11, doi: 10.2240/azojono0111.

Kawasaki E S and Player A. 2005. "Nanotechnology, nanomedicine, and the development of new, effective therapies for cancer." *Nanomedicine* 1: 101-109, doi: 10.1016/j.nano.2005.03.002.

Kim J H, Kim Y S, Park K, Lee S, Nam H Y, Min K H, Jo H G, Park J H, Choi K, Jeong S Y, Park R W, Kim I S, Kim K, Kwon I C. 2008.

Antitumor efficacy of cisplatin-loaded glycol chitosan nanoparticles in tumor-bearing mice. *J Control Release* 127: 41-49, doi: 10.1016/j.jconrel.2007.12.014.

Kim K S, Zhao Y, Jang H, Lee S Y, Kim J M, Kim K S, Ahn J H, Kim P, Choi J Y, Hong B H. 2009. "Large Scale Pattern Growth of Graphene Films for Stretchable Transparent Electrodes." *Nature* 457: 706-710, doi: 10.1038/nature07719.

Kohli A K and Alpar H O. 2004. "Potential use of nanoparticles for transcutaneous vaccine delivery: Effect of particle size and charge" *Int J Pharm* 275: 13-17, doi: 10.1016/j.ijpharm.2003.10.038.

Kopecek J, Kopeckova P. 2010. "HPMA copolymers: origins, early developments, present, and future." *Adv Drug Deliv Rev* 62: 122-149, doi: 10.1016/j.addr.2009.10.004.

Kreutera J, Petrov V E, Kharkevich D A, Alyautdin R N. 1997. "Influence of the type of surfactant on the analgesic effect induced by the peptide dalargin after its delivery across blood brain barrier using surfactant-coated nanoparticles." *J Control Rel* 49: 81, doi: 10.1016/S0168-3659(97)00061-8.

Kukowska-Latallo J F, Candido K A, Cao Z, Nigavekar S S, Majoros I J, Thomas T P, Balogh L P, Khan M K, Baker J R Jr. 2005. "Nanoparticle targeting of anticancer drug improves therapeutic response in animal model of human epithelial cancer." *Cancer Res* 65: 5317-5324, doi: 10.1158/0008-5472.CAN-04-3921.

Kumar P, Kulkarni P K, Srivastava A, Srivastava A. 2015. "Pharmaceutical application of nanoparticles in drug delivery system." *J Chem Pharm Res* 7: 703-712. http://www.jocpr.com/abstract/pharmaceutical-application-of-nanoparticles-in-drug-delivery-system-5650.html.

Kuppusamy P, Yusoff M M and Govindan N. 2014. "Biosynthesis of metallic nanoparticles using plant derivatives and their new avenues in pharmacological applications - An updated report." *Saudi Pharm. J* 24: 473-484, doi:10.1016/j.jsps.2014.11.013.

Lammers T, Ulbrich K. 2010. "HPMA copolymers: 30 years of advances." *Adv Drug Deliv Rev* 62: 119-121, doi: 10.1016/j.addr.2009.12.004.

Leroux J C, Allerman E, De Jaeghere F, Doelkar E, Gumy R. 1996. "Biodegradable nanoparticles -From sustained release formulations to improved site specific drug delivery" *J Cont Rel* 39: 339-350, doi: 10.1016/0168-3659(95)00164-6.

Li Y Z, Sun X, Gong T, Liu J, Zuo J, Zhaang Z R. 2010. "Inhalable microparticles as carriers for pulmonary delivery of thymopentin loaded solid lipid nanoparticles." *Pharm Res* 27: 1977-1986, doi: 10.1007/s11095-010-0201-z.

Lippacher A, Muller R H, Mader K. 2001. "Preparation of semisolid drug carriers for topical application based on solid lipid nanoparticles." *Int J Pharm* 214: 9–12, doi: 10.1016/S0378-5173(00)00623-2.

Liu Y, Miyoshi H and Nakamura M. 2007. "Nanomedicine for drug delivery and imaging: a promising avenue for cancer therapy and diagnosis using targeted functional nanoparticles." *Int. J. Cancer* 120: 2527-2537, doi: 10.1002/ijc.22709.

Lu C H and Jagannathan J. 2002. "Cerium-ion-doped yttrium aluminum garnet nanophosphors prepared through sol-gel pyrolysis for luminescent lighting." *Applied Physics Letters* 80: 3608-3610, doi: 10.1063/1.1475772.

Lu J, Shi M, Shoichet M S. 2009. "Click chemistry functionalized polymeric nanoparticles target corneal epithelial cells through RGD-cell surface receptors." *Bioconjug Chem* 20: 87-94, doi: 10.102 1/bc80031067.

Lugscheider E, Bärwulf S, Barimani C, Riester M and Hilgers H. 1998. "Magnetron-sputtered hard material coatings on thermoplastic polymers for clean room applications" *Surf Coatings Technol.* 108-109: 398–402, doi: 10.1016/S0257-8972(98)00627-6.

Mainardes R M, Urban M C, Cinto P O, Khalil N M, Chaud M V, Evangelista R C, Gremiao M P. 2005. "Colloidal carriers for ophthalmic drug delivery." *Curr Drug Targets* 6: 363-371, doi: 10.2174/1389450053765914.

Mittal G, Sahana D K, Bhardwaj V, Ravi Kumar M N. 2007. "Estradiol loaded PLGA nanoparticles for oral administration: effect of polymer molecular weight and copolymer composition on release behavior *in vitro* and *in vivo*" *J Control Rel* 119: 77-85, doi: 10.10/j.jconrel. 2007.01.016.

Morgan M T, Nakanishi Y, Kroll D J, Griset A P, Carnahan M A, Wathier M, Oberlies N H, Manikumar G, Wani M C, Grinstaff M W. 2006. "Dendrimer-encapsulated camptothecins: increased solubility, cellular uptake, and cellular retention afford enhanced anticancer activity *in vitro*." *Cancer Res* 66: 11913-11921, doi: 10.1158/0008-5472.CAN-06-2066.

Morita M, Rau D, Kajiyama S, Sakurai T, Baba M and Iwamura M. 2004. "Luminescence properties of nano-phosphors: metal-ion doped sol-gel silica glasses." *Materials Science-Poland* 22: 5-15. http://citeseerx.ist.psu.edu/viewdoc/download?doi=10.1.1.512.2884&rep=rep1&type=pdf.

Morones J R, Elechiguerra J L, Camacho A, Holt K, Kouri J B, Ramirez T J, Yacaman M J. 2005. "The bactericidal effect of silver nanoparticles." *Nanotechnology* 16: 2346-2353, doi: 10.1088/0957-4484/16/10/059.

Muller R H, Bohm B H L, Grau M J. 1999. "Nanosuspensions formulations for poorly soluble drugs with poor bioavailability: Stability, biopharmaceutical aspects possible drug forms and registration aspects." *Phram Ind* 61:175-178.

Muller R H, Keck C M. 2014. "Challenges and solutions for the delivery of biotech drugs – a review of drug nano crystal technology and lipid nanoparticles." *J Biotech* 113: 151-170, doi: 10.1016/j.jbiotec. 2004.06.007.

Nikula K, Snipes M, Barr E, Griffith W, Henderson R, Mauderly J. 1995. "Comparative pulmonary toxicities and carcinogenicities of chronically inhaled diesel exhaust and carbon black in F344 rats." *Fundam Appl Toxicol* 25: 80-94, doi: 10.1093/toxsci/25.1.80.

Nohynek G J, Schaefer H. 2001. "Benefit and risk of organic ultraviolet filters." *Regul Toxicol Pharmacol* 33: 285-291, doi: 10.1006/rtph.2001.1476.

Panyam J, Zhou W Z, Prabha S, Sahoo S K, Laabhasetwar B. 2002. "Rapid endo-lysosomal escape of poly(DL-lactide-co-glycolide) nanoparticles:

Implications for drug and gene delivery." *Faseb J* 16: 1217-1226, doi: 10.1096/fj.02-0088com.

Papakostas D; Rancan F; Sterry W; Annika V. 2011. "Nanoparticles in dermatology" *Arch Dermatol Res* 303: 533–550, doi: 10.1007/s00403-011-1163-7.

Park J, Fong P M, Lu J, Russell K S, Booth C J, Saltzman W M, Fahmy T M. 2009. "PEGylated PLGA nanoparticles for the improved delivery of doxorubicin." *Nanomedicine* 5: 410-418, doi: 10.1016/j.nano.200 9.02.002.

Patel M, Jain S K, Yadav A K, Gogna D, Agrawal G P. 2006. "Preparation and characterization of oxybenzone loaded gelatine microspheres for enhancement of sunscreeening efficacy." *Drug delivery* 13: 323-330, doi: 10.1080/10717540500398175.

Paul J, Borm A, Kreyling W. 2004. "Toxicological Hazards of Inhaled Nanoparticles- Potential Implications for Drug Delivery." *J Nanoscience Nanotechnol* 4: 1-11, doi: 10.1166/jnn.2004.081.

Pignatello R, Ricupero N, Bucolo C, Maugeri F, MalteseA, Puglisi G. 2006. "Preparation and characterization of Eudragit retard nanosuspensions for the o ular delivery of chloricomene" *AAPS Pharm Sci Tech* 7: 27, doi: 10.1208/pt070127.

Podaralla S, Sistla R, Saini T R, Diwan P V. 2006. "Influence of microencapsulation method and peptide loading on formulation of poly(lactide-co-glycolide) insulin nanoparticles" *Pharmazie* 61: 613-617, doi: 10.1007/0-387-27705-6_19.

Popov A P, Lademann J, Priezzhev A V, Myllyla R. 2005. "Effect of size of TiO_2 nanoparticles embedded into stratum corneum on ultraviolet-A and ultraviolet-B sun-blocking properties of the skin." *J Biomed Optics* 10: 1-9, doi: 10.1117/1.2138017.

Raghuvanshi R S, Katare Y K, Lalwani K, Ali M M, Singh O, Panda A K. 2002. "Improved immune response from biodegradable polymer particles entrapping tetanus toxoid by use of different immunization protocol and adjuvants." *Int J Pharm* 245: 109-121, doi: 10.1016/ S0378-5173(02)00342-3.

Rawat M, Singh D, Saraf S, Saraf S. 2006. "Nanocarriers: Promising Vehicle for Bioactive Drugs." *Biol Pharm Bull* 29: 1790-1798, doi: 10.1248/bpb.29.1790.

Safra T, Muggia F, Jeffers S, Tsao-Wei D D, Groshen S, Lyass O, Henderson R, Berry G, Gabizon A. 2000. "Pegylated ribosomal doxorubicin (doxil): reduced clinical cardiotoxicity in patients reaching or exceeding cumulative doses of 500mg/m." *Annal Oncol* 11: 1029-1033, doi: 10.1023/a:1008365716693.

Sajja H K, East M P, Mao H, Wang Y A, Nie S, Yang L. 2009. "Development of multifunctional nanoparticles for targeted drug delivery and non-invasive imaging of therapeutic effect." *Curr Drug Discov Technol* 6: 43-51, doi:10.2174/157016309787581066.

Salavati-niasari M, Davar F and Mir N. 2008. "Synthesis and characterization of metallic copper nanoparticles via thermal decomposition." *Polyhedron* 27: 3514-3518, doi: 10.1016/j.poly.2008.08.020.

Schinazi R F, Sijbesma R, Srdanov G, Hill C L, Wudl F. 1993. "Synthesis and Virucidal Activity of a Water-Soluble, Configurationally Stable, Derivatized C60 Fullerene." *Antimicrob Agents Ch* 37: 1707-1710, doi:10.1128/aac.37.8.1707.

Schroeder U, Sommerfeld P, Ulrich S, Sabel B A. 1998. "Nanoparticle technology for delivery of drugs across blood brain barrier." *J Pharm Science* 87: 1305-1307, doi: 10.1021/js980084y.

Shah P and Gavrin A Ã. 2006. "Synthesis of nanoparticles using high-pressure sputtering for magnetic domain imaging." *J Magn Magn Mater* 301: 118-123, doi: 10.1016/j.jmmm.2005.06.023.

Shim J, Kang H S, Park W S, Kim J, Chang I S. 2004. "Transdermal delivery of mixnoxidil with block copolymer nanoparticles." *J Control Rel* 97: 477-484, doi: 10.1016/j.jconrel.2004.03.028.

Singh S R, Grossniklaus H E, Kang S J, Edelhauser H F, Ambati B K, Kompella U B. 2009. "Intravenous transferrin, RGD peptide and dual-targeted nanoparticles enhance anti-VEGF intraceptor gene delivery to laser-induced CNV." *Gene Ther* 16: 645- 659, doi: 10.1038/gt.2008.185.

Son W K, Youk J H, Lee T S, Park W H. 2004. "Preparation of antimicrobial ultrafine cellulose acetate fibers with silver nanoparticles." *Macromol Rapid Commun* 25: 1632-1637, doi: 10.21002/marc.200400323.

Stober W, Fink A, Bohn E J. 1968. "Controlled growth of monodisperse silica spheres in the micron size range." *Colloid Interf Sci* 26: 62, doi:10.1016/0021-9797(68)90272-5.

Susa M, Iyer A K, Ryu K, Hornicek F J, Mankin H, Amiji M M, Duan Z. 2009. "Doxorubicin loaded Polymeric Nanoparticulate Delivery System to overcome drug resistance in osteosarcoma." *BMC Cancer* 9: 399-403, doi: 10.1186/1471-2407-9-399.

Tai C Y, Tai C, Chang M and Liu H. 2007. "Synthesis of Magnesium Hydroxide and Oxide Nanoparticles Using a Spinning Disk Reactor." *Ind Eng Chem Res* 46: 5536-5541, doi: 10.1021/ie060869b.

Torchilin V P. 2005. "Recent advances with liposomes as pharmaceutical carriers." *Nature Rev Drug Discov* 4: 145-160, doi: 10.1038/nrd1632.

Ulbrich K, Hekmatara T, Herbert E, Kreuter J. 2009. "Transferrin- and transferrinreceptor-antibody-modified nanoparticles enable drug delivery across the blood–brain barrier (BBB)." *Eur J Pharm Biopharm* 71: 251-256, doi: 10.1016/j.ejpb.2008.08.21.

Varde N K and Pack D W. 2004. "Microspheres for controlled release drug delivery." *Expert Opin Biol Ther* 4: 35-51, doi: 10.1517/ 14712598.4.1.35.

Vasir J K, Reddy M K, Labhasetwar V D. 2005. "Nanosystems in drug targeting: Opportunities and challenges." *Curr Nanosci* 1: 47-64, doi: 10.2174/1573413052953110.

Vijaykumar N, Venkateswarlu V, Raviraj P. 2012. "Drug nanoparticles-An overview" *Handbook on delivery of nanoparticles* 6: 111-132, doi: 10.5772/34680.

Vilaplana, J. L., Baeza, F. J., Galao, O., Zornoza, E., Garcés, P. 2013. "Self-sensing properties of alkali activated blast furnace slag (BFS) composites reinforced with carbon fibers." *Materials* 6: 4776-4786, doi: 10.3390/ma6104776.

Wang, J., Tian, S., Petros, R. A., Napier, M. E., Desimone, J. M. 2010. "The complex role of multivalency in nanoparticles targeting the transferrin receptor for cancer therapies." *J Am Chem Soc* 132: 11306-11313, doi: 10.1021/ja1043177.

Wang X, Li J, Wang Y, Cho KJ, Kim G, Gjyrezi A, Koenig L, Giannakakou P, Shin HJ, Tighiouart M, Nie S, Chen ZG, Shin DM (2009). HFT–T, a targeting nanoparticle, enhances specific delivery of paclitaxel to folate receptor-positive tumors. *ACS Nano* 3: 3165-74, doi: 10.1021/nn900649v.

Wangxi Z, Jie L, Gang W. 2003. "Evolution of structure and properties of PAN precursors during their conversion to carbon fibers." *Carbon* 41: 2805-2812, doi: 10.1016/S0008-6223(03)00391-9.

Wising S A, Muller R H. 2003. "Cosmetic application for solid lipid nanoparticles." *Int J Pharm* 254: 6-68, doi: 10.1016/S0378-5173(02)00684-1.

Wright C. 1997. "Micellar nanoparticle." US patent number 5, 620.021.

Wu F Y, Du J H, Liu C G, Li L X, Cheng H M. 2004. "The microstructure and energy storage characteristics of micro-coiled carbon fibers." *New Carbon Mater* 19: 81-86. http://en.cnki.com.cn/Article_en/CJFDTotal-XTCL200402001.htm.

Yadav N, Sunil K. 2013. "Solid lipid nanoparticles- A review" *Int J App Pharm* 5: 8-18. https://innovareacademics.in/journal/ijap/Vol5Issue2/111.pdf.

Yadav T P, Yadav R M and Singh D P. 2012. "Mechanical Milling: a Top Down Approach for the Synthesis of Nanomaterials and Nanocomposites." *Nanosci Nanotechnol* 2: 22-48, doi: 10.5923/j.nn.20120203.01.

Yamaguchi Y Nagasawa T, Nakamura N, Takenaga M, Mizoguchi M, Kawai S, Mizushima Y, Igarashi R. 2005. "Successful treatment of photodamaged skin of nano-scale at RA particles using novel transdermal delivery" *J Control Rel* 104: 29-40, doi: 10.1016/j.jconrel.2004.11.036.

Yu, Z. Q., Chang, D., Li, C., Zhang, N., Feng, Y. Y., and Dai, Y. Y. 2001. "Blue photoluminescent properties of pure nanostructured γ–Al2O3."

Material Research Society 16: 1890-1893, doi: 10.1557/JMR.2001.0259.

Zhang, L., Gu, F. X., Chan, J. M., Wang, A. Z., Langer, R. S., Farokhzad, O. C. 2008. "Nanoparticles in medicine: therapeutic applications and developments." *Clin. Pharmacol Ther* 83: 761-769, doi: 10.1038/sj.clpt.6100400.

Zhang Q, Shen Z, Nagai T. 2001. "Prolonged hypoglycemic effect of insulin-loaded polybutylcyanoacrylate nanoparticles after pulmonary administration to normal rats." *Int J Ph Parm* 218: 75-80, doi: 10.1016/S0378-5173(01)00614-7.

Zhang Z, Huey Lee S, Feng S S. 2007. "Folate-decorated poly(lactide-coglycolide)-vitamin E TPGS nanoparticles for targeted drug delivery." *Biomaterials* 28: 1889-1899, doi: 10.1016/j.biomaterials.2006.12.018.

In: Nanoparticles ISBN: 978-1-53616-596-8
Editors: A. K. Samantara, S. Ratha

Chapter 3

NANOMATERIALS AND CONJUGATES AS BIOMARKER: ADVANCED MATERIAL FOR *IN VITRO* AND *IN VIVO* CELL IMAGING

Alfa S. Mohanty*
Department of Botany, Regional Indtitute of Education,
Bhubaneswar, Odisha, India

ABSTRACT

Understanding of biological processes at the molecular level could bring significant progress in the evolution of diagnostic tools and innovative therapies. Fabrication of engineered nanomaterials is essential to enhance the next generation imaging technologies. Conventionally used imaging agents have few limiting factors such as low quantum yield, lack of *in vitro* and *in vivo* stability, insufficient photostability, low contrast sensitivity, poor spatial resolution and systemic cytotoxicity. In this context, nanomaterials like dye doped silica nanoparticles, graphene-based nanomaterials, magnetic nanoparticles, gold nanoparticles and quantum dots have been rigorously tested and have shown some intriguing properties that could help overcome many of such challenging

* Corresponding Author's Email: salfamohanty7@gmail.com.

issues and can be potential contenders for non-invasive bioimaging. However, integrating multimodal/multiplexed nanoparticles is a step forward to accomplish the increasing demand for dynamic bioimaging analysis with a focus on real-time and deep tissue penetrance through optical routes. This article illustrates the application of nanomaterials in live cell imaging including a brief background, synthesis/design protocols, modifications/functionalisation and physicochemical properties of nanomaterials along with major challenges and promising development in this domain.

Keywords: nanopartickes, imaging agents, quantum dots, contrasting agents, bioconjugates

1. INTRODUCTION

The first X-ray image was captured by Wilhelm Roentgen in 1896 of his wife's hand, which lead to a new era in medical diagnosis history. This discovery was then followed by the implementation of X-ray technology in different fields like bioimaging, drug delivery and clinical diagnosis. The visualization of internal body structures and visceral organs and tissues through bioimaging, enhanced the understanding process of organ functions. However, there are major obstacles in this field, such as different absorption coefficients of X-ray in tissues (Griffiths 1989, 202), near infrared absorption by fat tissues (Jacques 2013, 37) and imaging depths in different organs. These issues have propelled the rapid development of imaging modes to reveal the desired information by different stimuli, such as light, magnetic field, and ultrasound. Involvement of up-to-date technologies in the field of electronics, information technology, and more recently, nanotechnology, have provided significant push to the stimulated biomedical imaging. Substantial progress in the ability to fabricate and engineer particles in nanoscale and understanding of their unique physicochemical properties, have drawn significant attention from researchers (Murray 2000, 545). Development of contrast agents to selectively view specific biological events within the living system as well as the nonviable system has been made plausible, due to the advancement in bioimaging (Gui 2019, 82). However, targeted contrast agents with updated imaging modalities, engineered biomarkers and improved detection limits further added to better functionality of live cell imaging (Yin 2015, 4619). Inside the living system, some features do not need any contrast agent, for example, red blood cells can reflect ultrasound (Strohm & Kolios 2015, 741), and X-rays can be absorbed by the bones (Naumova 2014, 804). Contrast agents are essential for getting delicate images of fluids and structures with enhanced contrast. Conventional imaging techniques like computed tomography (CT), magnetic resonance imaging (MRI), positron emission tomography (PET), and single photon emission computed tomography (SPECT), have great imaging depths (Naumova 2014, 804). These imaging modes require functional organic molecules as contrast agents, e.g., barium/iodine in CT and radioactive tracers in PET. However, these molecular probes havecertain limitations; iodine/barium molecules have insufficient circulationtime (Cormode 2014, 37), radioactive fluorine-18 has short half-life (Sun 2011, 2999), and gadolinium ions and chelates have high levels oftoxicity (Ramalho 2016, 1192). Therefore, nanoprobes were modified for facile biofunctionalization and enhanced permeability and retention. Among the nanoprobes, optical nanoprobes were engineered for emissions and can be used for both fluorescent and luminescent imaging (FI & LI). The interior doped ions might also possess X-ray or magnetic properties.

Quantum yield and single excitation were shown by the nanoprobes based on CdSe photo luminescent (PL) semiconductor quantum dots (Bruchez 1998, 2013). But, high toxicity of Cd^{2+}, due to photo-oxidation under UV excitation (Derfus 2004, 11) and PL blinking drastically limit the quality of imaging (Efros & Nesbitt 2016, 661). The toxicity was suppressed by shallow penetration of UV and shell coating which was not applicable for *in vivo* studies (Anderson & Parrish 1981, 13). Microbubbles of diameter, 1-10 μm that are used in ultrasound imaging (USI), contain lipid shell, and protein/polymer encapsulating perfluorocarbon core. These help in large echogeneity for better ultrasound contrast (Anderson 2011, 215; Caskey 2007, 1191; Blomley 2001, 1222). In addition to that, shell materials can be modified for photoacoustic imaging (PAI) (Huynh 2012,

16464 ; Huynh 2014, 796). Although several attempts were made for bioimaging applications using different nanomaterials, the nanoprobes are unable to reach the tumor site for ultrasound imaging diagnosis due to the small sized pores in blood vessels at tumor site (Meng 2016, 8673). Recent studies have shown the extensive use of nanomaterials in imaging systems (Rieffel 2015, 4445; Smith & Gambhir 2017, 901; Li 2017, 1606857; Wang 2017, 6204 ; Lim 2015, 360; Gong 2017, 1393; Park 2017, 1600032). Some of the reports fascinated on single material system with broader scope. Therefore, this book chapter will provide a systematic and brief summary on the updated multifunctional bioimaging techniques with their applications. Frequently used imaging modes with their respective characteristic features are reviewed and discussed. Recently used nanomaterials which are in common use, i.e., lanthanide-ions-doped upconversion nanoparticles (UCNPs), carbon quantum dots (CQDs), echogenic nanobubbles (NBs), and derivatives of 2D materials have beendiscussed in details. Subsequently, different categories of engineered multimodal nanomaterials with their conjugates are discussed in brief with prototypical examples. Finally, best suitable candidates for bioimaging and suggestions on the future perspectives are presented which is expected to be essential for the development of new therapeutics.

2. Imaging Modalities

Nanomaterials are used in fluorescence, magnetic resonance, surface plasmon, Raman and surface enhanced Raman scattering (SERS), positron emission, photothermal and photo acoustic effects to solve various problems in medical and biological research like targeting biomolecules, drugs and imaging of sub-cellular organelles (Bodenmiller 2016, 225). The common imaging modes differ in respect to sensitivity, resolution, cost and data processing time, and each of these possess their respective features, advantages, and limitations (Liu 2015, 644). Choosing the appropriate imaging mode, completely depends on the specific query/concern that is to be addressed. Various optical imaging modes like MR (magnetic resonance), CT (computed tomography), PET (positron emission tomography) SPECT (single photon emission CT), US (ultrasound) and their subcategories and modified versions are also discussed (Huang 2015, 651). Imaging of biological specimens is dependent on both fluorescence and luminescence imaging, and have recently been updated due to technological advances. Consequently, MRI is mostly used in medical services for diagnosis of soft tissues. Subsequent advancement of imaging techniques by understanding their strength and weakness and synergistic effect of more than one modes for single system imaging is a step further in this direction. The combined effect of PET/CT permits to collect superciliousstructural and functional information of tissues/organs as well as integration of MRI/FI/SPECT allows to visualize the tissues inside (Madru 2014, 13). Fluorescence absorption and emission properties of the probes can be customized for improving penetration and resolution of *in vivo* optical images (Weissleder 2001, 316; Hong 2012, 1841), for example, mouse brain imaging have been carried outat more than 2 mm depth (Hong 2014, 723). However, trimodal imaging through upconversion luminescence (UCL)/MRI/CT allows bioimaging of internal tissue system through MRI/CT mode (Zeng 2012, 9232; Chen 2017, 5748). In this case, MRI/CT target organs and UCL imaging which was used for sensitive and planar resolution.

In this direction, apart from imaging modes, the nanoparticles were also exploited for their multimodal imaging properties. Hence, rapid fabrication of engineered nanomaterials and their intrinsic bioimaging properties further adds enhanced functionalities to bioimaging process. However, in some cases, surface modification of nanomaterials was required to immobilize the functional moieties for improved imaging needs. However, multimodal nanoparticles can be analysed by both magnetic resonance and optical imaging as in fluorescence microscopy. This is due to the generation of MRI signals in same particle by incorporating luminescent core and paramagnetic ions. These particles enhance the sensitivity and resolution of three dimensional imaging of cellular structures (Kayyem 1995, 615; Liang & Lauterbur 1994, 677). However, there are certain limitations such as limited anatomical background information of OI, and comparatively less sensitivity of MRI. This chapter willextent a concise review on the recent bioimaging techniques with a specific focus on designing nanomaterials for bioimaging and their applications.

Summary of imaging modes used in various applications are listed in Table 1. The basic principle of MRI relies on NMR (nuclear magnetic resonance). Through NMR, the hydrogen nuclei receives the signals generated from different tissues. Resonance was shown by nuclear spins at a specific frequency when a specimen lies in a static and homogenous magnetic field. Net magnetization changes when the specimen reaches its equilibrium magnetization and goes to an excited state. This excitation occurs at a proper resonant frequency with a radio frequency pulse. After the relaxation of spin, transmission of electromagnetic signals occurs to spectrophotometer. This difference in electromagnetic signals is used to build 3D images of the body. Brain and spinal cord lesions can be analysed using MRI due to its excellent soft tissue specificity. The major MRI parameters which influence the amount of signals are listed in Table 2 with the extent of contrast received from sample.

The values of the above parametersare responsible for contrast and are tissue specific, and can change from one to another. Contrast agents are injected to the patients due to the difficulties in distinguishing normal cell from tumor cell. Tumor cells can be selectively highlighted using contrast agents like iron particles, gadolinium chelates. Light is able to generate contrast by wavelength, intensity, polarization, interference, lifetime, coherence and nonlinear effects and is a versatile radiation for imaging. Many research group studied the interaction of light with various tissues (Alivisatos 2004, 47; Rudin 2005, 5; Weissleder 2006, 168; Ntziachristos 2009, 416).

Table 1. Summary of imaging modes

Imaging mode	Selected imaging system	Detection	Contrast agents	Application	Strengths	Weaknesses	References
CT	• Ionizing radiation • Low sensitivity	X-rays	Iopamidol, ioversol, iohexol, ioxaglate	Cerebral infarction, intracranial hemorrhage, angiography	Discovery CT750HD (GE Healthcare)	3D information available Relatively cheaper	Cheng 2014, 1886
MRI	SIGNA (GE Medical Systems)	Magnetic field	Gadoteridol, gadodiamide, gadopentetate dimeglumine	Cerebral and coronary angiography	Nonionizing Soft tissue imaging	Not suitable for patient with metallic implant Noisy	Chailangkarn 2016, 338
PET	Inveon (Siemens)	Gamma-rays	^{18}FDG, $^{15}H_2O$, ^{68}Ga-EDTA, 11C methionine	Cerebral blood flow and metabolic rates, degenerative diseases, brain development	Functional information of organs available	Low spatial resolution (≈1–2 mm) Shorter half-life of tracers (110 min for 18F)	Hedhli 2017, 3185 Pimlott & Sutherland. 2011, 149
SPECT	NanoSPECT/CT (Bioscan)	Gamma-rays	^{99m}Tc-HMPAO, ^{99m}Tc-ECD, 111In-octreotide	Cerebral infarction, ischemia, dementia, cardiac imaging	Cheaper than PET Longer half-life of tracers (up to tens of hours)	Low spatial resolution (≈1–2 mm) Long scan time	Pimlott & Sutherland. 2011, 149 Zhao 2016, 928

Table 2. Predominant factors influencing the signal from each location in MRI

Parameter	Description
T_1	Spin-lattice/longitudinal relaxation time. The T1 relaxation time constant is a material property describing the characteristics of how this energy is given back to the surroundings
T_2	Transverse relaxation time. T2relaxation time constant describes the energy transfer between adjacent protons
T_{2*}	Same as T2, but also contains heterogeneities in the environment
ρ	Spin density: the concentration of H nuclei in tissue

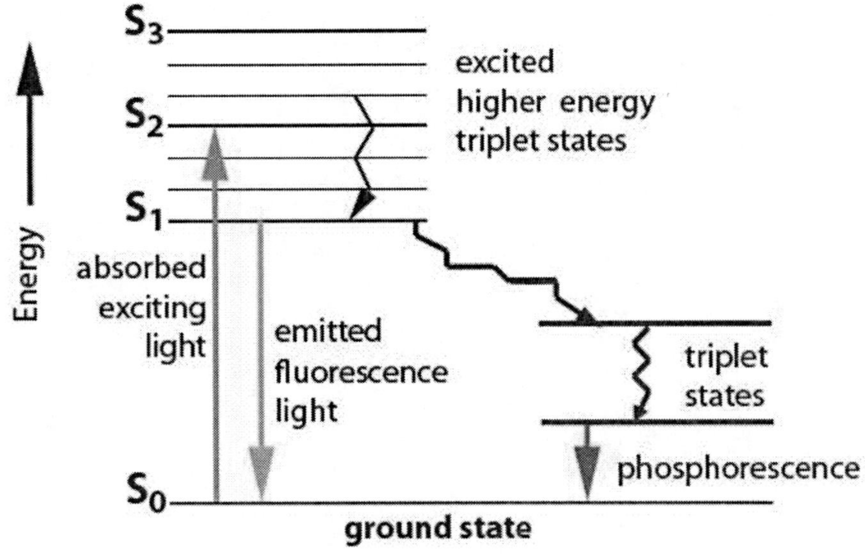

Figure 1. A Jablonski diagram.

Fluorescence is one of themost accepted optical imaging tools, which rely on fluorophore properties, i.e., organic dyes. Quanta of specific energy excite the fluorophore, which subsequently excites electrons from ground state to a higherenergy singlet state like S1, S2 (Figure 1). Energy carried by electrons can be of different types like vibrational and rotational. The conversion to a singlet state requires shift to an equivalent rotational or vibrational energy. The electron loses its energy by thermal decay, resulting emission of lower energy photon. Fluorescence requires a difference in excitation and emission wavelengths. While the fundamental barrier includes autofluorescence, high light scattering and high absorption can be found in the case of hemoglobin. Different penetration depths can be obtained depending on the wavelength of light irradiated (Table 3). Therefore, NIR source of wavelengths ranging between 650-900 nm can achieve higher penetration of tissue in comparison to UV-visible spectral range. This is mainly due to the reduction of absorbance from tissue surface in the respective spectral regions.

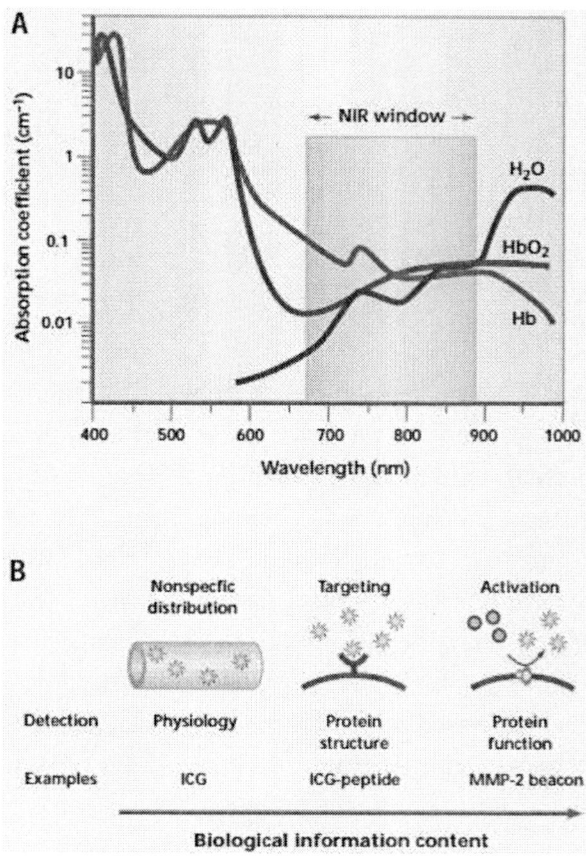

Figure 2. The NIR window is ideally suited for *in vivo* imaging because of minimal light absorption by hemoglobin (< 650 nm) and water (> 900 nm) (Weissleder 2001, 316).

Table 3. Optical imaging techniques

Technique	Depth	Commonly used wavelength	Clinical potential
Microscopic resolution			
Epi A	20 μm	Visible	Experimental
Confocal	500 μm	Visible	Experimental
Two-photon	800 μm	Visible	Yes
Mesoscopic resolution			
Optical projection tomography	15 mm	Visible	No
Optical coherence tomography	2 mm	Visible, NIR	Yes
Laser speckle imaging	1 mm	Visible, NIR	Yes
Macroscopic resolution, intrinsic contrast			
Hyperspectral imaging	< 5 mm	Visible	Yes
Endoscopy	< 5 mm	Visible	Yes
Polarization imaging	< 1.5 cm	Visible, NIR	Yes
Fluorescence reflectance imaging	< 7 mm	NIR	Yes
Diffuse optical tomography	< 20 cm	NIR	Yes
Macroscopic resolution, molecular contrast			
Fluorescence resonance imaging	< 7 mm	NIR	Yes
Fluorescence molecular tomography	< 20 cm	NIR	Yes
Bioluminescence imaging	< 3 cm	500–600 nm	No

Hemoglobin is a primary absorber of visible light while water and lipid are absorber of infrared light (Licha 2001, 44). They have the lowest absorption coefficients in the NIR region (Weissleder 2001, 316) (Figure 2). Thus, deeper areas allow tomographic images of bulk tissue. Updated fluorescence imaging techniques like FMT and FRI utilize NIR wavelengths for bioimaging of living tissues (Ntziachristos 2004, 12294; Weissleder & Ntziachristos 2003, 123; Ntziachristos 2002, 1535350020 0201121; Gremlich 2004, 15353500200404127). As studied by Weissleder group, FMT and FRI based probe detected breast cancers and distinguished it from the normal cells (Bremer 2005, 321327). IVM is a powerful technique, which uses fluorescent probes to analyze molecular process. IVM permits extended monitoring of living tissues in cellular and molecular processes with the resolution of 1-10 μm (Jain 2003, 685; Jain 2007, 610).

3. IMAGING AGENTS

Imaging agents can be divided into following two broad categories as discussed follows,

3.1. Endogenous Agents

Enzymes are used to mediate the process within the physiological system, which generate the visible light for degrading the substance. In this direction, the fluorescent proteins such as green fluorescent protein (GFP) (Gurskaya 2001, 16; Labas 2002, 4256; Yanushevich 2005, 43; Gurskaya 2006, 461) and luciferase bioluminescence are employed as reporter system. Again (Burch 2005, 995; Gade 2005, 9080; Zhao 2005, 041210; Villalobos 2005, 131), GFP proteins can be used for long-term measurements due to their less photoleaching property (Hoffman & Yang 2005, 790), and they don't require further substrates to perform. During synthesis, the protein is covalently attached to the fluorescent pigment (Matz 2002, 953). Ultimately, the gene expression associated with GFP directly leads to green fluorescent signal, determined by mature protein position. GFP can be used for extracting information from cellular and molecular level (Kishimoto 2013, 79453; Li 2017, 1606857), but certain drawbacks like low emission wavelength (λ= 510nm) overlapping autofluorescence in tissues limits their role in clinical applications. To overcome some issues faced during the use of endogenous fluorophores, bioluminescence can be used. Mostly, luciferin is used as a substrate in bioluminescence and administered to organisms carrying luciferase enzyme. They make enzyme substrate complex, which oxidizes the luciferase. Oxidised luciferase emits light which is detected for analysis. The promising application of bioluminescence is limited, due to stable luciferase expression, issues with light penetration and positional uncertainty of light emitting cells, because of non-homologous scattering.

3.2. Exogenous Imaging Agents

Exogenous imaging agents ranging from dyes to fluorescent probes serve as most appreciable contrast agents for bioimaging applications now-a-days; for example, gadolinium chelates and super paramagnetic iron oxide are used in MRI, lanthanide chelates and organic fluorophores used in fluorescence imaging. However, there are a number of limitations associated with their implementation. In the following section, nanomaterials' involvement in solving the issues regarding the contrast agents is discussed in details.

3.3. Conventional Contrast Agents

3.3.1. Organic Dyes

Most commonly used fluorophores in biological applications include organic fluorescent dyes such as fluorescein isothiocyanate (FITC) and carboxyfluorescein diacetate succinimidyl ester (CFSE). These are used to stain cell organelles by (Lyons & Paris 2005, 3165) labeling antibodies and biomolecules. However, they are associated with certain limitations like,

(i) They cannot be used for prolonged bioimaging analysis due to rapid photo bleaching (inability to fluoresce continuously for a long time) (Akerman 2002, 12617).
(ii) Local chemical environment like pH, ionic medium, etc. strongly influence the emission and excitation processes.
(iii) Multicolor imaging is not possible for organic fluorophores, due to relatively broad emission spectrum overlapping with emission of other fluorophores. Excitation of each fluorophore occurs by photon sources.
(iv) Tissues give small amount of auto fluorescence due to the presence of fluorophores like elastin, collagen, flavins, and nicotinamides. These tissue level auto fluorescence can overlap with the emission of most of the dyes by giving background fluorescence in the same

visible region. To overcome this, cyanide class of fluorochrome dyes are employed exogenously which fluoresce in near infrared region (Ntziachristos & Chance 2000, 41; Tung 2004, 391; Pham 2004, 1403). Most of the conventional dyes which emit light beyond ~850 nm suffer from poor photostability, and low brightness/quantum yield (Bhushan 2004, 17648; Kim 2007, 7661).

3.3.2. MRI Contrast Agents

Paramagnetic properties shown by some of the transition metals and lanthanide series metals make them good candidate for MRI contrasting agents, as these materials enhance contrast via alteration of local magnetic environment by facilitating T_1 and T_2 relaxation process. Gd(III) is one of the widely accepted contrast agents due to its larger magnetic field. DTPA (diethyltriaminepentaacetic acid) is a chelating group thatusually binds to Gd(III) ion forming GD-DTPA, is also well appreciated for imaging applications. Besides the above mentioned points, some practical issues are there which need to be considered:

(i) Among the frequently used MRI contrast agents, the uptake potential was limited in the case of Gd-DTPA due to rapid non-specific equilibration between intraand extravascular space.
(ii) Ionic form of Gd is toxic, having a half-life of several weeks. Its stability was influenced during administration by parameters such as pH, temperature and concentration of ions and ligands. Again, Gd can be displaced by endogenous metals like Cu and Zn, from the complex. Demetallation was observed in bones and liver with the deposition of Gd(III) ion by Weinmann et al. Moreover, issues with time were observed with Gd chelates during contrast enhanced MRI, dose dependent performance in patients with tumors of CNS, surgically induced contrast enhancement leads to unnecessary resection due to confusion with residual tumor enhancement (Sieber 2008, 65). Apart from these, gadolinium chelate based MRI contrast enhancement faces the difficulties with

time and dose (Knauth 2001, 254; Franiel. 2008, 481) and surgically induced contrast enhancement, which was resulted due to surgical manipulation (Wirtz 2000, 1112; Schneider 2005, 489). This sometimes leads to unnecessary resection due to confusion with residual tumor enhancement. Iron oxide, as magnetic nanoparticle, has evolved as an MRI contrast agent (Weissleder 1995, 321 ; Kircher 2003, 8122) for liver and spleen. But, higher toxicity of magnetic nanoparticles restricts their use in human beings.

3.4. Nanoparticle-Based Contrast Agents

The key features, which must be kept in mind while using a fluorescence based optical imaging agent, are as follows:

(i) Stability in *in vivo* and *in vitro* systems;
(ii) Resistance to photobleaching;
(iii) Higher absorbance and quantum yield;
(iv) Non-toxicity and resistivity for metabolic disintegration;
(v) NIR range emission (700–900 nm) and
(vi) Requisite dispersibility in themedium.

As free Gd is known to be toxic, it is important to have it in complex or in permanently chelated form. The essential requirements that need to be considered while designing Gd(III) chelates as MRI contrast agents are thermal stability, synthesis and kinetics (Comblin 1999, 451; Woods 2005, 3829). Targeted sequestration of imaging agent is the most important part to limit the toxicity raised due to non-specific uptake of contrast agents. Recently reported nanoparticle based exogenous contrast agents include gold nanoparticles, organically modified silica, lanthanide derivatives, etc. possess all of the aforementioned desired features.

3.5. Dye-Doped Silica Nanoparticles

As discussed above, rapid photobleaching is one of the major issues with organic fluorescent dyes. Photodegradation of dye have been observed in the cellular environment (Song 1996, 2959; Jaiswal 2003, 47). *In vitro* and *in vivo* stability of dye can be maximized by encapsulating it in a ceramic matrix. Different techniques that are in use for the process of encapsulation include incorporation of the sample in nucleic acid and PNA oligomers lipid micelles polymer matrices and encapsulation in silica matrix (Tapec 2002, 405; Zheng 2002, 1485; Lian 2004, 135; He 2004, 585; Ye 2005, 51; Bagwe 2006, 4357; Wang 2008, 99). This minimizes oxygen access, increases chemical stability and allows surface modification of the shell to enhance hydrophilic character and cell uptake.

3.5.1. Basis of Optical Detection

The chief source of fluorescence is the 'dye' encapsulated within the matrix of the nanoparticles. The fluorescence emission can be altered marginally after encapsulation with some added advantages. Encapsulation of dye effectively suppresses rapid photobleaching (Rosi 2006, 1027), by preventing it from being exposed directly to the surrounding chemicals. A novel fluorescence lifetime-based approach to determine the core-shell structure of the dye (fluorescein isothiocyanate) doped silica nanoparticle have been reported, which revealed that approximately 62% of dye molecules remained in the solvated silica shell, while 38% of dye molecules remained in the non-solvated (dry) silica core. This permits the imaging process to be performed over extended period of time.

3.5.2. Properties

There are several reasons for which silica coated particles are preferred as biomarkers:

(i) Amorphous silica has beenfound to have excellent biocompatibility (Lytton-Jean & Mirkin 2005, 12754) and is a non-toxic (Smith 2002, 54) material.

(ii) The interaction potential achieved by theouter shells of silica coated particles drastically influences the aggregation behavior.

(iii) During encapsulation, spectral characteristics were not altered and remained intact. Silica particle provides a protective layer and can entrap fluorescent dyes inside it (Van Blaaderen, & Vrij 1992, 2921). Protection is mainly due to the reduction of penetration in oxygen molecule resulting into photodegradation of dye molecule. Dye degradation occurs in both air and water (in this case, dissolved oxygen). As a result, photostability of silica coated dye molecules is higher than that of bare dye, in solution.

(iv) Matrix of silica is optically transparent due to which emission and excitation light can pass through efficiently.

(v) Change in solvent polarity does not affect the size of silica particles and silica porosity due to swelling resistance. Therefore, wide varieties of solvents can be used during encapsulation.

(vi) There are several methods available to encapsulate the dye. For example, modified stober's method can be used to attach the dye to silica or encapsulation can be done in reverse micellar medium.

(vii) Conventional silane based chemistry can be used for surface modification of silica particles for the attachment of biomolecules (Qhobosheane 2004, 635) such aspeptides, protein, nucleotides, antibodies, etc. For example, cysteine containing peptides can be adhered to the aminated silica nanoparticles and stable covalent amide bond can be formed between carboxylated silica nanoparticles and amine groups of proteins and antibodies (Bera 2010, 2260).

3.6. Quantum Dots

Quantum Dots (QDs) are semiconductor crystals andused preferably as biomarkers, because they will overlap some drawbacks of organic dyes. They luminesce due to quantum confinement effects. Oneof the very first examples of QDs, being usedas luminescence probes in cell imaging, has been reported by Alivisatos and Nie's groups. After that, there has been a significant increase in the use of these quantum dots for bioimaging. In many cases, these luminescent particles behave like a transitional stage between single atom and bulk semiconductor. However, quantum mechanical effects wereshown by electrons by these size arrangements (Steigerwald & Brus 1990, 183; Weller 1993, 88; Weller 1993, 41; Cherepy 1998, 770; Weller 1998, 194; Gaponenko, S.V. 1998; Michler 2000, 968).

3.6.1. Spectral Properties

(i) By altering the size and elemental composition of QD core, we can change the emission spectra from UV (blue) to NIR (Mattoussi et al. 2000). QDs emitting in similar region are gaining importance due to emission and excitation of probes in NIR range.
(ii) QDs are suitable for the detection of biological samples, as the emission and excitation spectra are favorable. Their emission spectra are narrow and excitation spectra are broad, which helps to reduce the overlapping of spectra, subsequently improving the differentiation of multiple fluorophore.

3.6.2. Resistance to Photobleaching

The alteration of molecular structure of dye due to the absorption of excitation light, leads to permanent loss of its fluorescence properties, called photobleaching. In the case of QDs, the photostability comes from the shell surrounding the core.

3.6.3. Resistance to Metabolic Degradation

In addition to other properties, the QDs' inorganic nature and their protective coatings also influence the resistance to various metabolic degradations. Cell viability study was carried out by treating a frog with QDsat different stages of development starting from embryo to tadpole stage (Dubertret 2002, 1759). This report confirms the nontoxicity of coated QDs with all normal phenotypes.

3.6.4. High Extinction Coefficients

QDs resultin bright fluorescent probes due to higher quantum yield and molar extinction coefficients (Akerman 2002, 12617). Their molar extinction coefficientsare of the order of $0.5 - 5 \times 10^{-6}$ M^{-1} cm^{-1} (Steckel 2004, 1862). This resulted inhigh brightness in in-vivo circumstances (light intensities decreased due to absorption and scattering) and in aqueous solutions. However, conjugation with other biomolecules has noeffect on the quantum yield (Qu 2001, 333).

3.6.5. Conjugation Ability

A number of methods can be used for bioconjugation of QDs, e.g., conjugating them with linkers such as protein A or protein G, avidin, or a secondary antibody (Goldman 2002, 6378) through covalent binding (Dubertret 2002, 1759), electrostatic interaction, multivalent chelation and passive adsorption. Most of the proteins have amine and carboxylic groups as their functional groups, so surface functionalization by amide cross-linking is the most frequent tool to carry out the bioconjugation process.

4. Designing Nanoparticles for Bioimaging

Design of nanomaterials is the most important step of bioimaging study and certain points should be kept in mind during the designing and fabrication of nanomaterials. They are detailed in the following points.

(i) Synthesis of optical core: Core formation is the 1st step towards synthesis. The core encapsulates fluorochome, e.g., dyes or quantum dots. Among the micro-emulsion methods used, "water-in-oil" (w/o) technique is by far the most popular method for nanoparticle fabrication by micro-emulsion system. This is commonly referred as the reverse micelles and has broad range of scopes for alteration of reaction conditionsby optimizing the concentration, oil, temperature, composition of polar media, ratio of surfactant and co-surfactant for nanoparticle designing. Some books are available which have provided detailed discussions on this specific topic (Finean1883, 225; Rosano & Clausse 1987; Pileni 1989, 302; Kumar & Mittal 1999).

(ii) Synthesis of shell: Optical core is protected by the shell from the surrounding environment, which enhances the optical properties due to thelattice mismatch with the quantum dots, giving additional photostability to organic dyes. This also provides binding ability to themolecules for bioconjugation and surface stability.

(iii) Surface modification: Coagulation and aggregation are the two natural phenomena observed in the case of most of these nanostructured particles. In an aqueous environment, nanoparticles should be uniformly dispersed to be used for any application. Surface modification of nanomaterials with dispersing agents and polymers, etc. could solve this problem to a large extent.

(iv) Bioconjugation and targeting: While using nanoparticles for bioimaging, desirable delivery of functionalized materials to the target site of action has always been a key concern. Most of the times, biomolecules like peptides, amines, antibodies, enzymes, etc. get attached to the nanomaterials for targeted binding and promote dispersion too. Drug and nanoparticle conjugation can be achieved by both active and passive processes. In the case of active targeting, surface modification of nanomaterials iscarried out with molecules those are having affinity towards the targeted cells (Bala 2004, 387), and in the case of passive targeting, accumulation of drug or drug carrier system is triggered at a particular site of interest, due to physicochemical or pharmacological factors (Vasir 2005, 47; Gindy 2009, 65).

During the fabrication of nanosytems for optical bioimaging, all of the aforementioned points need to be taken care of. A detailed discussion on the design and fabrication of dye-doped nanoparticles and gold nanoparticles with their properties have been provided in the following section.

4.1. Dye-Doped Silica Nanoparticles

4.1.1. Optical Core

Major preparatory methods of silica nanoparticles include microemulsion mediated method (Esquena. 1997, 6400; Arriagada & Osseo-Asare 1999, 210; Osseo-Asare & Arriagada1999, 68), and the sol-gel process (Klein1988) (i.e., Stober's method) (Stober 1968, 62). While in a typical Stober's method, alkoxysilane compounds (e.g., tetraethyl orthosilicate (TEOS), tetramethyl orthosilicate (TMOS) and their derivatives, etc.) undergo base catalyzed hydrolysis and condensation reaction in ammonia–ethanol–water mixture, similar reaction can also take place in the microemulsion system core. Several kinds of silica nanoparticles (SiNPs) were studied for sensing and imaging (Burns 2006, 723; Wang 2013, 1367). PEGylated mesoporous and fluorescent SiNPs with a single pore have shown good results (Schreml 2014, 721). Now-a-days, mesoporous SiNPs are used extensively, because of their ability to incorporate heavy dye loading. They can also be synthesized and functionalized using hydrothermal reactions. Dye is encapsulated within a silica shell in the case of dye doped silica nanoparticles, and this can be done by either covalent attachment of the dye with silica precursors like APTS before the hydrolysis in Stober's method or by solubilising the dye in the microemulsioncore followed by polymerization (Bagwe 2006, 4357). Stober's method has advantage over microemulsion because of the scaling ability for synthesis of nanoparticles, and the yield is comparatively much higher. Certain drawbacks of this techniqueinclude varied particle sizes and difficulty in achieving surface modification. But, synthesis using microemulsion method moreover gives uniform particles and permits easy surface tunability.

4.1.2. Shell Synthesis

Microemulsion is the most commonly used method (i.e., TMOS/ TEOS), for coating of the core by further condensation of the silane reagents.

4.1.3. Surface Modification

For bioconjugation, shell formation can be done by carboxyl derivatives or amine derivatives like APTS. Other compounds can be used to prevent agglomeration of nanoparticles in aqueous medium. Dispersion can be achieved instantly using controlled amount of APTS, TEOS, etc.

4.1.4. Bioconjugation

Carboxyl functionalized nanoparticle can be attached covalently to carboxyl containing biomolecules like peptides, amines, enzymes, etc. through carbodiimide coupling chemistry (Paulos et al. 2004).

Nanoparticles, such as dye-doped fluorescent silica nanoparticles, having inbuilt fluorescence properties are used in fluorescent labeling method, as has been proposed by He et al. (He 2004, 585). Nanoparticles, synthesized using microemulsion w/o method, can selectively identify the target cell. They are covalently immobilized with Hab18 (antihuman liver cancer monoclonal antibody) which recognizes HepG liver cancer cells. During the operation of various fluorescence labeling techniques, ultrasensitive detection from target can be achieved by the combination of high-intensity luminescent particles and antibody. In the same manner, reverse micelle based synthesis of SiO_2 composite particles modified with chitosan have been used for DNA labeling. There are a broad range of examples of SiNPs based bioimaging techniques, because of the ability of SiNPs to accommodate fluorescent/MRI/PET/SPECT contrast agents, and it is easier to modulate the pore or surface of these nanoparticles with gene/drug molecule (Yoon 2006, 209). Fluorescent probes like fluorescein isothiocyanate, rhodamine isothiocyanate, cyanine dyes, methyl violegen, alexafluor dyes, coordination complexes of ruthenium, terbium and europium, and semiconductor quantum dots can be conjugated to SiNPs and delivered or injected efficiently to different cell lines (Reiter 2007, 3680).

4.2. Gold Nanoparticles

Gold nanoparticles have been used as coloring agents since few decades. Their size and shape dependent physiochemical properties including Surface Plasmon Resonance (SPR) imparts uniqueness and distinguishes them from others in wide areas of applications like sensing, catalysis, solar energy harvesting, photothermal therapy and drug delivery. Properties of gold nanoparticles primarily rely on their shape, size, dispersive index and surface chemistry. The craze of gold nanoparticle was perceived after the introduction of monodispersed colloidal gold with citrate duringthe latter half of 20th century. Afterwards, several fruitful modifications have been achieved by different groups. Biphasic synthesis by Shiffrin Brust got popularity due to the involvement of simple steps and reagents (Brust 1994, 801).

4.2.1. Optical Core Synthesis

As we have already discussed, colorimetric contrast of nanosized gold is due to SPR. SPR is a function of size, shape and dielectric constant of the medium. A number of preparatory methods have been established, which mechanistically based on the reduction of precursor gold ions in the presence of reducing agents, microemulsions, through radiation techniques, surfactants, seed mediated method, copolymer micelles, etc. (Palmal & Jana 2014, 102).

4.2.2. Surface Modification

Surface functionalization is a major step to improve dispersion and to allow bioconjugation for optical imaging.

4.2.3. Bioconjugation

Electrostatic interaction is a key factor behind the adherence of a positively charged biomolecule like protein to a negatively charged gold nanoparticle or sulphohydryl group can participate in bond formation because of their high efficiency towards gold atoms (Giersig & Mulvaney 1993, 3408). Thiol oligonucleotide coated gold nanoparticle in biological buffers has been reported by Mirkin's group (Elghanian 1997, 1078). Signal was provided by the molecules present in the gap between two consecutive molecules of gold nanocrystals (Jiang 2003, 9964). Hence, ligand exchange reaction and surface modification are two key factors for adapting gold nanosystems for bioimaging applications. The unique properties of gold nanosystems which made them more useful in optical imaging field are biocompatibility, SPR tuning capability, and photodecomposition.

4.3. Quantum Dots (QDs)

A number of unique properties possessed by the quantum dots make them an appropriate candidate as bioimaging agent; large surface area, stable and bright photoluminescence, broad absorption and narrow emission bands and large one and two photon absorption cross-sections, for the *in vitro* and *in vivo* detection/imaging of biomolecules, cells and tissues.

4.3.1. Optical Core Synthesis

Several reviews have covered the synthesis and preparation of semiconductor nanoparticles (Green 2005, 3002). Metal precipitation in the presence of colloidal stabilizers is one of the preparation methods for QDs like Hg, Cd, Zn and the hydroxides of Se, S, etc. (Dung 1988, 2977 ; Rossetti & Brus 1988, 4470). Afterwards, a more convenient method used for synthesis involves high temperature of 300°C. High temperature facilitates the synthesis of highly crystalline QDs with high quantum yields. And, the presence of a surfactant prevents agglomeration and provides space for crystal growth, limit dissolution of small crystals through Ostwald ripening. 'Water in oil' microemulsion or reverse micellar method also is a frequently used method for the preparation of QDs, which involves metal and chalcogenide precipitation in water, yielding nanocrystals coated with surfactant. Some of the examples of QDs prepared with this w/o microemulsions method are CdS, CdMnS, ZnSe, etc. (Kobayashi 2001, 1630; Karanikolos 2004, 550; Pang 2004, 213).

4.3.2. Shell Synthesis

In the previous section covering details about the resistance in photobleaching, we have discussed that a shell comprising a large band gap semiconductor covered the core. For example, the core of CdSe QDs was covered by the epitaxially matched ZnS layer, effectively passivating the surface defects of CdSe, and preventing photo-corrosion. This is the major cause of quantum yield enhancement. Capping can be done with ZnSe (Hoener et al. 1992).

4.3.3. Surface Modification

A surface capping of organic ligand monolayer was found in TOPO based nanocrystals. They are soluble in nonpolar solvents. Amphiphilic polymers like PEG help in the dispersion of these hydrophobic dots and reduce nonspecific adhesion. Other polymer may result in blockage of copolymer and polyanhydride. The surfaces of the QDs were also protected by silica layer. QDs of best quality can be synthesized in organic phase through highly hydrophobic aliphatic ligand ssuch as alkyl phosphines, alkyl phosphine oxides, aliphatic amines and aliphatic carboxylic acids. Therefore, ligand exchange reactions and surface modifications have become necessary for biological applications of quantum dots.

4.3.4. Bioconjugation

Surface chemistry of QDs are designed to facilitate reactive functional groups for direct conjugation to biomolecules like amine ($-NH_2$), carboxyl (–COOH) or mercapto (–SH) groups. Finally, the QDs are conjugated to the linker (e.g., avidin, protein A or protein G, or a secondary antibody) by covalent binding passive adsorption, multivalent chelation or by electrostatic interactions (discussed above, in the conjugation ability section). One of the simplest protocols for the covalent conjugation of quantum dots with biomolecules is EDC coupling. For example, the carboxylic acid group in thioglycolic acid or dihydrolipoic acid functionalized quantum dots can be conjugated with amino groups in biomolecules such as peptides, proteins, antibodies or DNA by EDC coupling. Here, the possible complexity associated with cross-linking among multiple carboxyl and amino groups present in most biomolecules should be carefully considered and minimized.

CONCLUSION

Diversification in the use of nanomaterials is due primarily to the unique properties they carry endogenously, along with a large number of physical and chemical methods of preparation. In addition to that, appropriate surface functionalization can make them a suitable candidate for multimodal imaging. However, selection of nanomaterials for fluorescent imaging is one of the most difficult steps to get desirable outcome. Nanomaterials can be used in both extracellular and intracellular analysis and depending on the application, nanomaterials can be chosen. During the selection, few critical factors are to be taken into consideration; nontoxic and cell permeable bright particles are suitable for plain imaging, e.g., mesoporous silica, upconversion nanocrystals, etc. Targeted imaging requires surface modification with ligands for receptors. Biocompatibility is a major factor, while imaging carried out with biosystems. Optical and multimodal imaging demand sophisticatedly designed nanomaterials, which are expected to give bright fluorescence, and can incorporatefunctional materials inside the core or shell without any alteration of physicochemical properties. Some particles were designed with porous shell for loading with photothermal/photodynamic agent, drug or a gene. Further, the release of drug or gene at target site is a matter of concern. Therefore, a number of issues such as toxicity, biocompatibility, bio availability *in vivo* and *in vitro* targeting efficiency, renal and hepatobiliary clearance of functionalized nanoprobes are under extreme investigation. Light, temperature and pH optimization can solve the issues of controlled release. Nevertheless, construction of nanomaterials by differential conjugation methods with genes, drugs, targeting molecules, contrast agents have been extensively studied for treatment of diseases. However, clinical application of nanomaterial formulation is significantly hindered due to some controversial outputs related to both toxicity and pharmacokinetics.

Progress has been made in bioimaging with the implementation of nuclear techniques like PET, SPECT, and fluorescent probes. More sensitivity of imaging can be achieved with the use of near-IR fluorochromes, coupled with fluorescence enhanced tomography. Organic dyes are mostly hydrophobic and their fluorescence quenched in isotonic solution. To overcome these limitations, nanomaterials were introduced, but the use of nanomaterials does not solve the issue completely. Some major points must be taken into consideration during fluorophore based clinical translation, i.e., photostability, optimization of loading dye, detection of fluorescent signals from interior target organs and suitable probes having narrow symmetric emission spectrum. Irreversible aggregation exhibited by gold nanostructures in the presence of inappropriate buffers is due to their sensitivity towards ionic strength and pH of medium or surface passivation. Almost all thenanoprobes can be purified with centrifugation;however, purification of synthesized and functionalized carbon quantum dots is a tedious task, as it involves membrane filtering, dialysis and gel columns for down streaming of probes for bioimaging. Lanthanum (Ln^{3+}) based UCNPs was found to have excellent optical and physiochemical properties which makes it an appropriate choice as nanoprobe, but the quantum yield in this case remains 5% lesser than CQDs. Bioimaging might be affected by large distributions of large particles, as they cannot enter targeted sites of small cellular structures. Among the bioimaging nanomaterials, derivatives of 2D materials are the most recently used ones, but their immune response, long term toxicity, clearance and feasibility for clinical diagnosis are yet to be studied. Despite the vast advancement of computational and analytical techniques, toxicity is still a matter of concern in the case of nanomaterials and it's difficult to generalize. Hence, preclinical studies which can contribute to the nanoprobes database for future safety assessment are prerequisite for multimodal bioimaging. Recent studies include imaging with long-term tracking with the involvement of persistent luminescence, NIR laser and X –ray for rechargeable imaging and long-term or extended monitoring with X-ray, etc. Hence, in addition to in-depth studies of existing nanoprobes, the search for new non-toxic, biocompatible and dischargeable nanosystems with outstanding contrast ability should be continued.

References

Akerman, M. E., Chan, W. C., Laakkonen, P., Bhatia, S. N. & Ruoslahti, E. (2002). "Nanocrystal targeting *in vivo*." *Proceedings of the National Academy of Sciences*, *99*, 12617-12621. doi: 10.1073/pnas.152463399.

Alivisatos, P. (2004). "The use of nanocrystals in biological detection." *Nature biotechnology*, *22*, 47.doi:10.1038/nbt927.

Anderson, C. R., Hu, X., Tlaxca, J., Decleves, A. E., Houghtaling, R., Sharma, K. & Rychak, J. J. (2011). "Ultrasound molecular imaging of tumor angiogenesis with an integrin targeted microbubble contrast agent." *Investigative radiology*, *46*, 215.doi: 10.1097/ RLI.0b013e3182 034fed.

Anderson, R. R. & Parrish, J. A. (1981). "The optics of human skin." *Journal of investigative dermatology*, *77*, 13-19. doi: 10.1111/ 1523-1747.ep12479191

Arriagada, F. J. & Osseo-Asare, K. (1999). "Synthesis of nanosize silica in a nonionic water-in-oil microemulsion: effects of the water/surfactant molar ratio and ammonia concentration." *Journal of colloid and interface science*, *211*, 210-220.doi: 10.1006/jcis.1998.5985.

Bagwe, R. P., Hilliard, L. R. & Tan, W. (2006). "Surface modification of silica nanoparticles to reduce aggregation and nonspecific binding." *Langmuir*, *22*, 4357-4362. doi: org/10.1021/la052797j.

Bala, I., Hariharan, S. & Kumar, M. R. (2004). "PLGA nanoparticles in drug delivery: the state of the art." *Critical Reviews™ in Therapeutic*

Drug Carrier Systems, *21*, 387-422.doi: 10.1615/ CritRevTherDrug CarrierSyst.v21.i5.20.

Bera, D., Qian, L., Tseng, T. K. & Holloway, P. H. (2010). "Quantum dots and their multimodal applications: a review. *Materials*, *3*, 2260-2345. doi: 10.3390/ma3042260.

Bhushan, K. R., Misra, P., Liu, F., Mathur, S., Lenkinski, R. E. & Frangioni, J. V. (2008). "Detection of breast cancer microcalcifications using a dual-modality SPECT/NIR fluorescent probe." *Journal of the American Chemical Society*, *130*, 17648-17649. doi: 10.1021/ ja807099s.

Blomley, M. J., Cooke, J. C., Unger, E. C., Monaghan, M. J. & Cosgrove, D. O. (2001). "Microbubble contrast agents: a new era in ultrasound." *Bmj*, *322*, 1222-1225. doi:10.1136/bmj.322.7296.1222.

Bodenmiller, B. (2016). "Multiplexed epitope-based tissue imaging for discovery and healthcare applications." *Cell systems*, *2*, 225-238. doi: 10.1016/j.cels.2016.03.008.

Bremer, C., Ntziachristos, V., Weitkamp, B., Theilmeier, G., Heindel, W. & Weissleder, R. (2005). "Optical imaging of spontaneous breast tumors using protease sensing 'smart' optical probes." *Investigative radiology*, *40*, 321-327.doi: 10.1097/01.rli.0000163797.23172.90.

Bruchez, M., Moronne, M., Gin, P., Weiss, S. & Alivisatos, A. P. (1998). "Semiconductor nanocrystals as fluorescent biological labels." *Science*, *281*, 2013-2016. doi: 10.1126/science.281.5385.2013.

Brust, M., Walker, M., Bethell, D., Schiffrin, D. J. & Whyman, R. (1994). "Synthesis of thiol-derivatised gold nanoparticles in a two-phase liquid–liquid system." *Journal of the Chemical Society, Chemical Communications*, *7*, 801-802.doi: 10.1039/C39940000801.

Burch, S., Bisland, S. K., Bogaards, A., Yee, A. J. M., Whyne, C. M., Finkelstein, J. A. & Wilson, B. C. (2005). "Photodynamic therapy for the treatment of vertebral metastases in a rat model of human breast carcinoma." *Journal of orthopaedic research*, *23*, 995-1003. doi: 10.1016/j.orthres.2004.12.014

Burns, A., Sengupta, P., Zedayko, T., Baird, B. & Wiesner, U. (2006). Core/shell fluorescent silica nanoparticles for chemical sensing:

towards single-particle laboratories. *Small*, *2*, 723-726. doi: 10.1002/smll.200600017.

Caskey, C. F., Stieger, S. M., Qin, S., Dayton, P. A. & Ferrara, K. W. (2007). "Direct observations of ultrasound microbubble contrast agent interaction with the microvessel wall." *The Journal of the Acoustical Society of America*, *122*, 1191-1200. doi: 10.1121/1.2747204.

Chailangkarn, T., Trujillo, C. A., Freitas, B. C., Hrvoj-Mihic, B., Herai, R. H., Diana, X. Y. & Stefanacci, L. (2016). "A human neurodevelopmental model for Williams syndrome." *Nature*, *536*, 338. doi:10.1038/nature19067

Chen, C., Liu, J., Chen, Y., Li, C., Liu, X., Huang, H. & Feng, S. (2017). "Sub-10 nm Sr2LuF7: Yb/Er@ Sr2GdF7@ SrF2 Up-Conversion Nanocrystals for Up-Conversion Luminescence–Magnetic Resonance–Computed Tomography TrimodalBioimaging." *ACS applied materials & interfaces*, *9*, 5748-5756. doi: 10.1021/acsami.6b14007.

Cheng, L., Liu, J., Gu, X., Gong, H., Shi, X., Liu, T. & Bu, W. (2014). "PEGylated WS2 nanosheets as a multifunctional theranostic agent for *in vivo* dual-modal CT/photoacoustic imaging guided photothermal therapy." *Advanced materials*, *26*, 1886-1893. doi:10.1002/adma.201304497

Cherepy, N. J., Liston, D. B., Lovejoy, J. A., Deng, H. & Zhang, J. Z. (1998). "Ultrafast studies of photoexcited electron dynamics in γ-and α-Fe2O3 semiconductor nanoparticles." *The Journal of Physical Chemistry B*, *102*, 770-776. doi: 10.1021/jp973149e.

Comblin, V., Gilsoul, D., Hermann, M., Humblet, V., Jacques, V., Mesbahi, M. & Desreux, J. F. (1999). "Designing new MRI contrast agents: a coordination chemistry challenge." *Coordination chemistry reviews*, *185*, 451-470. doi:10.1016/S0010-8545(99)00028-4.

Cormode, D. P., Naha, P. C. & Fayad, Z. A. (2014). "Nanoparticle contrast agents for computed tomography: a focus on micelles." *Contrast media & molecular imaging*, *9*, 37-52. doi: 10.1002/cmmi.1551.

Derfus, A. M., Chan, W. C. & Bhatia, S. N. (2004). "Probing the cytotoxicity of semiconductor quantum dots." *Nano letters*, *4*, 11-18. doi: 10.1021/nl0347334.

Dubertret, B., Skourides, P., Norris, D. J., Noireaux, V., Brivanlou, A. H. & Libchaber, A. (2002). "*In vivo* imaging of quantum dots encapsulated in phospholipid micelles." *Science*, *298*, 1759-1762. doi: 10.1126/science.1077194.

Dung, D., Ramsden, J. & Graetzel, M. (1982). "Dynamics of interfacial electron-transfer processes in colloidal semiconductor systems." *Journal of the American Chemical Society*, *104*, 2977-2985. doi: 10.1021/ja00375a006.

Efros, A. L. & Nesbitt, D. J. (2016). "Origin and control of blinking in quantum dots." *Nature nanotechnology*, *11*, 661. doi: 10.1038/ NNA NO.2016.140.

Elghanian, R., Storhoff, J. J., Mucic, R. C., Letsinger, R. L. & Mirkin, C. A. (1997). "Selective colorimetric detection of polynucleotides based on the distance-dependent optical properties of gold nanoparticles." *Science*, *277*, 1078-1081. doi: 10.1126/science.277.5329.1078.

Esquena, J., Tadros, T. F., Kostarelos, K. & Solans, C. (1997). "Preparation of narrow size distribution silica particles using microemulsions." *Langmuir*, *13*, 6400-6406. doi: 10.1021/la9705120.

Finean, J. B. (1983). "Membrane mimetic chemistry—characterization and applications of micelles, microemulsions, monolayers, bilayers, vesicles, host-guest systems, and polyions." *Trends in Biochemical Sciences*, *8*, 225. doi:10.1016/0968-0004(83)90225-6.

Franiel, T., Lüdemann, L., Rudolph, B., Rehbein, H., Staack, A., Taupitz, M. & Beyersdorff, D. (2008). "Evaluation of normal prostate tissue, chronic prostatitis, and prostate cancer by quantitative perfusion analysis using a dynamic contrast-enhanced inversion-prepared dual-contrast gradient echo sequence." *Investigative radiology*, *43*, 481-487. doi: 10.1097/RLI.0b013e31816b2f63.

Gade, T. P., Hassen, W., Santos, E., Gunset, G., Saudemont, A., Gong, M. C. & Lyddane, C. (2005). "Targeted elimination of prostate cancer by genetically directed human T lymphocytes." *Cancer research*, *65*, 9080-9088. doi: 10.1158/0008-5472.

Gaponenko, S. V. (1998). "*Optical properties of semiconductor nanocrystals*," (Vol. *23*). Cambridge university press.

Giersig, M. & Mulvaney, P. (1993). "Preparation of ordered colloid monolayers by electrophoretic deposition." *Langmuir*, *9*, 3408-3413. doi: 10.1021/la00036a014.

Gindy, M. E. & Prud'homme, R. K. (2009). "Multifunctional nanoparticles for imaging, delivery and targeting in cancer therapy." *Expert opinion on drug delivery*, *6*, 865-878. doi: 10.1517/17425240902932908.

Goldman, E. R., Balighian, E. D., Mattoussi, H., Kuno, M. K., Mauro, J. M., Tran, P. T. & Anderson, G. P. (2002). "Avidin: a natural bridge for quantum dot-antibody conjugates." *Journal of the American Chemical Society*, *124*, 6378-6382. doi: 10.1021/ja0125570.

Gong, L., Wang, Y. & Liu, J. (2017). "Bioapplications of renal-clearable luminescent metal nanoparticles." *Biomaterials science*, *5*, 1393-1406. doi: 10.1039/C7BM00257B.

Green, M. (2005). "Organometallic based strategies for metal nanocrystal synthesis." *Chemical communications*, *24*, 3002-3011. doi: 10.1039/B501835H.

Gremlich, H. U., Martinez, V., Kneuer, R., Kinzy, W., Weber, E., Pfannkuche, H. J. & Rudin, M. (2004). "Noninvasive assessment of gastric emptying by near-infrared fluorescence reflectance imaging in mice: pharmacological validation with tegaserod, cisapride, and clonidine." *Molecular imaging*, *3*, 15353500200404127. doi: 10.1162/15353500200404127.

Griffiths, H. J. (1989). "Tissue Substitutes in Radiation Dosimetry and Measurement." No. 4. *Radiology*, *173*, 202-202. doi: 10.1148/radiology.173.1.202.

Gui, R., Jin, H., Bu, X., Fu, Y., Wang, Z. & Liu, Q. (2019). "Recent advances in dual-emission ratiometric fluorescence probes for chemo/biosensing and bioimaging of biomarkers." *Coordination Chemistry Reviews*, *383*, 82-103. doi: 10.1016/j.ccr.2019.01.004.

Gurskaya, N. G., Fradkov, A. F., Terskikh, A., Matz, M. V., Labas, Y. A., Martynov, V. I. & Lukyanov, S. A. (2001). "GFP-like chromoproteins as a source of far-red fluorescent proteins." *FEBS letters*, *507*, 16-20.doi:10.1016/s0014-5793(01)02930-1.

Gurskaya, N. G., Verkhusha, V. V., Shcheglov, A. S., Staroverov, D. B., Chepurnykh, T. V., Fradkov, A. F. & Lukyanov, K. A. (2006). "Engineering of a monomeric green-to-red photoactivatable fluorescent protein induced by blue light." *Nature biotechnology*, *24*, 461. doi:10.1038/nbt1191.

He, L., Musick, M. D., Nicewarner, S. R., Salinas, F. G., Benkovic, S. J., Natan, M. J. & Keating, C. D. (2000). "Colloidal Au-enhanced surface plasmon resonance for ultrasensitive detection of DNA hybridization." *Journal of the American Chemical Society*, *122*, 9071-9077. doi:10.1021/ja001215b.

He, X., Duan, J., Wang, K., Tan, W., Lin, X. & He, C. (2004). "A novel fluorescent label based on organic dye-doped silica nanoparticles for HepG liver cancer cell recognition." *Journal of nanoscience and nanotechnology*, *4*, 585-589. doi:10.1166/jnn.2004.011.

Hedhli, J., Czerwinski, A., Schuelke, M., Płoska, A., Sowinski, P., La Hood, L. & Dobrucki, I. T. (2017). "Synthesis, chemical characterization and multiscale biological evaluation of a dimeric-cRGD peptide for targeted imaging of α v β 3 integrin activity." *Scientific reports*, *7*, 3185. doi:10.1038/s41598-017-03224-8.

Hoffman, R. M. & Yang, M. (2005). "Dual-color, whole-body imaging in mice." *Nature biotechnology*, *23*, 790. doi:10.1038/nbt0705-790.

Hong, G., Diao, S., Chang, J., Antaris, A. L., Chen, C., Zhang, B. & Kuo, C. J. (2014). "Through-skull fluorescence imaging of the brain in a new near-infrared window." *Nature photonics*, *8*, 723. doi:10.1038/nphoton.2014.166.

Hong, G., Lee, J. C., Robinson, J. T., Raaz, U., Xie, L., Huang, N. F. & Dai, H. (2012). "Multifunctional *in vivo* vascular imaging using near-infrared II fluorescence." *Nature medicine*, *18*, 1841. doi:10.1038/nm.2995.

Huang, C. L., Huang, C. C., Mai, F. D., Yen, C. L., Tzing, S. H., Hsieh, H. T. & Chang, J. Y. (2015). "Application of paramagnetic graphene quantum dots as a platform for simultaneous dual-modality bioimaging and tumor-targeted drug delivery." *Journal of Materials Chemistry B*, *3*, 651-664. doi:10.1039/c4tb01650e.

Huynh, E., Jin, C. S., Wilson, B. C. & Zheng, G. (2014). "Aggregate enhanced trimodalporphyrin shell microbubbles for ultrasound, photoacoustic, and fluorescence imaging." *Bioconjugate chemistry*, *25*, 796-801. doi: 10.1021/bc5000725.

Huynh, E., Lovell, J. F., Helfield, B. L., Jeon, M., Kim, C., Goertz, D. E. & Zheng, G. (2012). "Porphyrin shell microbubbles with intrinsic ultrasound and photoacoustic properties." *Journal of the American Chemical Society*, *134*, 16464-16467. doi:10.1021/ja305988f.

Jacques, S. L. (2013). "Optical properties of biological tissues: a review." *Physics in Medicine & Biology*, 58: R37. doi:10.1088/0031-9155/58/11/r37.

Jain, R. K. (2003). "Molecular regulation of vessel maturation. *Nature medicine*, *9*, 685. doi:10.1038/nm0603-685.

Jain, R. K., Di Tomaso, E., Duda, D. G., Loeffler, J. S., Sorensen, A. G. & Batchelor, T. T. (2007). "Angiogenesis in brain tumours." *Nature Reviews Neuroscience*, *8*, 610. doi:10.1038/nrn2175.

Jaiswal, J. K., Mattoussi, H., Mauro, J. M. & Simon, S. M. (2003). "Long-term multiple color imaging of live cells using quantum dot bioconjugates." *Nature biotechnology*, *21*, 47. doi:10.1038/nbt767.

Jiang, J., Bosnick, K., Maillard, M. & Brus, L. (2003). "Single molecule Raman spectroscopy at the junctions of large Ag nanocrystals." *The Journal of Physical Chemistry B*, *107*, 9964–9972. doi:10.1021/jp034632u.

Karanikolos, G. N., Alexandridis, P., Itskos, G., Petrou, A. & Mountziaris, T. J. (2004). "Synthesis and Size Control of Luminescent ZnSe Nanocrystals by a Microemulsion−Gas Contacting Technique." *Langmuir*, *20*, 550-553. doi:10.1021/la035397.

Kayyem, J. F., Kumar, R. M., Fraser, S. E. & Meade, T. J. (1995). "Receptor-targeted co-transport of DNA and magnetic resonance contrast agents." *Chemistry & biology*, *2*, 615-620. doi:10.1016/1074-5521(95)90126-4.

Kim, D., Park, S., Lee, J. H., Jeong, Y. Y. & Jon, S. (2007). "Antibiofouling polymer-coated gold nanoparticles as a contrast agent for *in vivo* X-ray computed tomography imaging." *Journal of the*

American Chemical Society, *129*, 7661-7665. doi:10.1016/ j.nano.2007.10.072.

Kircher, M. F., Mahmood, U., King, R. S., Weissleder, R. & Josephson, L. (2003). "A multimodal nanoparticle for preoperative magnetic resonance imaging and intraoperative optical brain tumor delineation." *Cancer research*, *63*, 8122-8125.

Kishimoto, H., Momiyama, M., Aki, R., Kimura, H., Suetsugu, A., Bouvet, M. & Hoffman, R. M. (2013). "Development of a clinically-precise mouse model of rectal cancer." *PloS one*, *8*, e79453. doi:10.1371/ journal.pone.0079453.

Klein, L. C. (1988). "Text book of Sol-Gel technology for thin films, fibers, performs, electronics, and specialty shapes.

Knauth, M., Wirtz, C. R., Aras, N. & Sartor, K. (2001). "Low-field interventional MRI in neurosurgery: finding the right dose of contrast medium." *Neuroradiology*, *43*, 254-258. doi:10.1007/pl00006047.

Kobayashi, Y., Salgueirino-Maceira, V. & Liz-Marzán, L. M. (2001). "Deposition of silver nanoparticles on silica spheres by pretreatment steps in electroless plating." *Chemistry of Materials*, *13*, 1630-1633. doi:10.1021/cm001240g.

Kumar, P. & Mittal, K. L. (Eds.). (1999). *Handbook of microemulsion science and technology*. CRC press.

Labas, Y. A., Gurskaya, N. G., Yanushevich, Y. G., Fradkov, A. F., Lukyanov, K. A., Lukyanov, S. A. & Matz, M. V. (2002). "Diversity and evolution of the green fluorescent protein family." *Proceedings of the National Academy of Sciences*, *99*, 4256-4261. doi:10.1073/ pnas.062552299.

Li, X., Kim, J., Yoon, J. & Chen, X. (2017). "Cancer-associated, stimuli-driven, turn on theranostics for multimodality imaging and therapy." *Advanced Materials*, *29*, 1606857. doi:10.1002/ adma.201606857.

Lian, W., Litherland, S. A., Badrane, H., Tan, W., Wu, D., Baker, H. V. & Jin, S. (2004). "Ultrasensitive detection of biomolecules with fluorescent dye-doped nanoparticles." *Analytical biochemistry*, *334*, 135-144. doi:10.1016/j.ab.2004.08.005.

Liang, Z. P. & Lauterbur, P. C. (1994). "Efficient magnetic resonance imaging using a generalized series model." *IEEE Trans Med Imaging*, *13*, 677-686. doi: 10.1109/42.363100.

Licha, K., Hessenius, C., Becker, A., Henklein, P., Bauer, M., Wisniewski, S. & Semmler, W. (2001). "Synthesis, characterization, and biological properties of cyanine-labeled somatostatin analogues as receptor-targeted fluorescent probes." *Bioconjugate chemistry*, *12*, 44-50. doi:10.1021/bc000040s.

Lim, S. Y., Shen, W. & Gao, Z. (2015). "Carbon quantum dots and their applications." *Chemical Society Reviews*, *44*, 362-381. doi:10.1039/c4cs00269e.

Liu, Z., Lavis, L. D. & Betzig, E. (2015). "Imaging live-cell dynamics and structure at the single-molecule level." *Molecular cell*, *58*, 644-659. doi:10.1016/j.molcel.2015.02.033.

Lyons, A. B. & Parish, C. R. (1995). "Are murine marginal-zone macrophages the splenic white pulp analog of high endothelial venules?" *European journal of immunology*, *25*, 3165-3172. doi:10.1002/eji.1830251127 .

Lytton-Jean, A. K. & Mirkin, C. A. (2005). "A thermodynamic investigation into the binding properties of DNA functionalized gold nanoparticle probes and molecular fluorophore probes." *Journal of the American Chemical Society*, *127*, 12754-12755. doi:10.1021/ja052255o.

Madru, R., Svenmarker, P., Ingvar, C., Ståhlberg, F., Engels, S. A., Knutsson, L. & Strand, S. E. (2014). "Development of a hybrid nanoprobe for triple-modality MR/SPECT/optical fluorescence imaging." *Diagnostics*, *4*, 13-26. doi:10.3390/diagnostics4010013.

Matz, M. V., Lukyanov, K. A. & Lukyanov, S. A. (2002). "Family of the green fluorescent protein: journey to the end of the rainbow." *Bioessays*, *24*, 953-959. doi:10.1002/bies.10154.

Meng, M., Gao, J., Wu, C., Zhou, X., Zang, X., Lin, X. & Wang, Y. (2016). "Doxorubicin nanobubble for combining ultrasonography and targeted chemotherapy of rabbit with VX2 liver tumor." *Tumor Biology*, *37*, 8673-8680. doi:10.1007/s13277-015-4525-5.

Michler, P., Imamoğlu, A., Mason, M. D., Carson, P. J., Strouse, G. F. & Buratto, S. K. (2000). "Quantum correlation among photons from a single quantum dot at room temperature." *Nature*, *406*, 968. doi:10.1038/35023100.

Murray, C. B., Kagan, A. C. & Bawendi, M. G. (2000). "Synthesis and characterization of monodisperse nanocrystals and close-packed nanocrystal assemblies." *Annual review of materials science*, *30*, 545-610. doi:10.1146/annurev.matsci.30.1.545.

Naumova, A. V., Modo, M., Moore, A., Murry, C. E. & Frank, J. A. (2014). "Clinical imaging in regenerative medicine." *Nature biotechnology*, *32*, 804. doi:10.1038/nbt.2993.

Ntziachristos, V. (2009). "Optical imaging of molecular signatures in pulmonary inflammation." *Proceedings of the American Thoracic Society*, *6*, 416-418. doi:10.1513/pats.200901-003aw.

Ntziachristos, V. & Chance, B. (2000). "Breast imaging technology: Probing physiology and molecular function using optical imaging-applications to breast cancer." *Breast Cancer Research*, *3*, 41. doi:10.1186/bcr269.

Ntziachristos, V., Bremer, C., Graves, E. E., Ripoll, J. & Weissleder, R. (2002). "*In vivo* tomographic imaging of near-infrared fluorescent probes." *Molecular Imaging*, *1*, 15353500200201121. doi:10.1162/15353500200201121.

Ntziachristos, V., Schellenberger, E. A., Ripoll, J., Yessayan, D., Graves, E., Bogdanov, A. & Weissleder, R. (2004). "Visualization of antitumor treatment by means of fluorescence molecular tomography with an annexin V–Cy5. 5 conjugate." *Proceedings of the National Academy of Sciences*, *101*, 12294-12299. doi:10.1073/pnas.0401137101.

Osseo-Asare, K. & Arriagada, F. J. (1999). "Growth kinetics of nanosize silica in a nonionic water-in-oil microemulsion: a reverse micellarpseudophase reaction model.: *Journal of colloid and interface science*, *218*, 68-76. doi: 10.1006/jcis.1999.6232.

Palmal, S. & Jana, N. R. (2014). "Gold nanoclusters with enhanced tunable fluorescence as bioimaging probes." *Wiley Interdisciplinary Reviews:*

Nanomedicine and Nanobiotechnology, *6*, 102-110. doi:10.1002/ wnan.1245.

Pang, Q., Guo, B. C., Yang, C. L., Yang, S. H., Gong, M. L., Ge, W. K. & Wang, J. N. (2004). "Cd1− xMnxS quantum dots: new synthesis and characterization." *Journal of crystal growth*, *269*, 213-217. doi:10.1016/j.jcrysgro.2004.04.119.

Park, J. E., Kim, M., Hwang, J. H. & Nam, J. M. (2017). "Golden opportunities: Plasmonic gold nanostructures for biomedical applications based on the second near-infrared window." *Small Methods*, *1*, 1600032. doi:10.1002/smtd.201600032.

Pham, W., Choi, Y., Weissleder, R. & Tung, C. H. (200)4. "Developing a peptide-based near-infrared molecular probe for protease sensing." *Bioconjugate chemistry*, *15*, 1403-1407. doi:10.1021/ bc049924s.

Pileni, M. P. (1989). "Structure and reactivity in reverse micelles." *Analytica Chimica Acta*, *242*, 302–303. doi:10.1016/0003-2670(91)87089-p.

Pimlott, S. L. & Sutherland, A. (2011). "Molecular tracers for the PET and SPECT imaging of disease." *Chemical Society Reviews*, *40*, 149-162. doi:10.1039/b922628c.

Qhobosheane, M., Zhang, P. & Tan, W. (2004). "Assembly of silica nanoparticles for two-dimensional nanomaterials." *Journal of nanoscience and nanotechnology*, *4*, 635-640. doi:10.1166/ jnn. 2004.014.

Qu, L., Peng, Z. A. & Peng, X. (2001). "Alternative routes toward high quality CdSe nanocrystals." *Nano Letters*, *1*, 333-337.doi:10.1021/ nl0155532

Ramalho, J., Semelka, R. C., Ramalho, M., Nunes, R. H., AlObaidy, M. & Castillo, M. (2016). "Gadolinium-based contrast agent accumulation and toxicity: an update." *American Journal of Neuroradiology*, *37*, 1192-1198. doi:10.3174/ajnr.a4615.

Rieffel, J., Chitgupi, U. & Lovell, J. F. (2015). "Recent advances in higher-order, multimodal, biomedical imaging agents." *Small*, *11*, 4445-4461. doi:10.1002/smll.201500735.

Rieter, W. J., Kim, J. S., Taylor, K. M., An, H., Lin, W., Tarrant, T. & Lin, W. (2007). "Hybrid silica nanoparticles for multimodal imaging." *Angewandte Chemie International Edition*, *46*, 3680-3682. doi:10.1002/ange.200604738.

Rosano, H. L. & Clausse, M. (Eds.). (1987). *Microemulsion systems*, (Vol. *24*). CRC Press.

Rosi, N. L., Giljohann, D. A., Thaxton, C. S., Lytton-Jean, A. K., Han, M. S. & Mirkin, C. A. (2006). "Oligonucleotide-modified gold nanoparticles for intracellular gene regulation." *Science*, *312*, 1027-1030. doi:10.1126/science.1125559.

Rossetti, R. & Brus, L. (1982). "Electron-hole recombination emission as a probe of surface chemistry in aqueous cadmium sulfide colloids." *The Journal of Physical Chemistry*, *86*, 4470-4472. doi:10.1021/j100220a003.

Rudin, M., Rausch, M. & Stoeckli, M. (2005). "Molecular imaging in drug discovery and development: potential and limitations of nonnuclear methods." *Molecular Imaging and Biology*, *7*, 5-13. doi:10.1007/s11307-004-0954-z.

Schneider, J. P., Trantakis, C., Rubach, M., Schulz, T., Dietrich, J., Winkler, D. & Zimmer, C. (2005). "Intraoperative MRI to guide the resection of primary supratentorialglioblastomamultiforme—a quantitative radiological analysis." *Neuroradiology*, *47*, 489-500. doi:10.1007/s00234-005-1397-1.

Schreml, S., Meier, R. J., Kirschbaum, M., Kong, S. C., Gehmert, S., Felthaus, O. & Albert, M. (2014). "Luminescent dual sensors reveal extracellular pH-gradients and hypoxia on chronic wounds that disrupt epidermal repair." *Theranostics*, *4*, 721. doi:10.1016/ j.nhtm. 2014.11.052.

Sieber, M. A., Pietsch, H., Walter, J., Haider, W., Frenzel, T. & Weinmann, H. J. (2008). "A preclinical study to investigate the development of nephrogenic systemic fibrosis: a possible role for gadolinium-based contrast media." *Investigative radiology*, *43*, 65-75. doi:10.1097/rli.0b013e31815e6277.

Smith, B. R. & Gambhir, S. S. (2017). "Nanomaterials for *in vivo* imaging." *Chemical reviews*, *117*, 901-986. doi: 10.1021/ acs.chemrev.6b00073.

Smith, P. W. (2002). "Fluorescence emission-based detection and diagnosis of malignancy." *Journal of Cellular Biochemistry*, *87*, 54-59. doi:10.1002/jcb.10403.

Song, L., Varma, C. A., Verhoeven, J. W. & Tanke, H. J. (1996). "Influence of the triplet excited state on the photobleaching kinetics of fluorescein in microscopy." *Biophysical journal*, *70*, 2959-2968. doi:10.1016/ s0006-3495(96)79866-1.

Steckel, J. S., Coe-Sullivan, S., Bulović, V. & Bawendi, M. G. (2003). "1.3 μm to 1.55 μm tunable electroluminescence from PbSe quantum dots embedded within an organic device." *Advanced Materials*, *15*, 1862-1866. doi:10.1002/adma.200305449.

Steigerwald, M. L. & Brus, L. E. (1990). "Semiconductor crystallites: a class of large molecules." *Accounts of Chemical Research*, *23*, 183-188. doi:10.1021/ar00174a003.

Stober, W., Fink, A. & Bohn, E. (1968). "Controlled growth of monodisperse silica spheres in the micron size range." *Journal of colloid and interface science*, *26*, 62-69. doi:10.1016/0021-9797(68)90272-5.

Strohm, E. M. & Kolios, M. C. (2015). "Classification of blood cells and tumor cells using label-free ultrasound and photoacoustics." *Cytometry Part A*, *87*, 741-749. doi:10.1002/cyto.a.22698.

Sun, Y., Yu, M., Liang, S., Zhang, Y., Li, C., Mou, T. & Li, F. (2011). "Fluorine-18 labeled rare-earth nanoparticles for positron emission tomography (PET) imaging of sentinel lymph node." *Biomaterials*, *32*, 2999-3007. doi:10.1016/j.biomaterials.2011.01.011.

Tapec, R., Zhao, X. J. & Tan, W. (2002). "Development of organic dye-doped silica nanoparticles for bioanalysis and biosensors." *Journal of nanoscience and nanotechnology*, *2*, 405-409. doi:10.1166/ jnn.2002.114.

Tung, C. H. (2004). "Fluorescent peptide probes for *in vivo* diagnostic imaging." *Peptide Science: Original Research on Biomolecules, 76*, 391-403. doi:10.1002/bip.20139.

Van Blaaderen, A. & Vrij, A. (1992). "Synthesis and characterization of colloidal dispersions of fluorescent, monodisperse silica spheres." *Langmuir, 8*, 2921-2931. doi:10.1021/la00048a013.

Vasir, J. K., Reddy, M. K. & Labhasetwar, V. D. (2005). "Nanosystems in drug targeting: opportunities and challenges." *Current Nanoscience, 1*, 47-64. doi:10.2174/1573413052953110.

Villalobos, C., Nadal, A., Núñez, L., Quesada, I., Chamero, P., Alonso, M. T. & García-Sancho, J. (2005). "Bioluminescence imaging of nuclear calcium oscillations in intact pancreatic islets of Langerhans from the mouse." *Cell Calcium, 38*, 131-139. doi:10.1016/j.ceca.2005.06.029.

Wang, J., Ma, Q., Wang, Y., Shen, H. & Yuan, Q. (2017). "Recent progress in biomedical applications of persistent luminescence nanoparticles." *Nanoscale, 9*, 6204-6218. doi:10.1039/c7nr01488k.

Wang, K., He, X., Yang, X. & Shi, H. (2013). "Functionalized silica nanoparticles: a platform for fluorescence imaging at the cell and small animal levels." *Accounts of chemical research, 46*, 1367-1376. doi:10.1021/ar3001525.

Wang, L., Zhao, W. & Tan, W. (2008). "Bioconjugated silica nanoparticles: development and applications." *Nano Research, 1*, 99-115. doi:10.1007/s12274-008-8018-3.

Weissleder, R. (2001). "A clearer vision for *in vivo* imaging." *Nature Biotechnology, 19*, 316–317. doi:10.1038/86684.

Weissleder, R. (2006). "Molecular imaging in cancer." *Science, 312*, 1168-1171. doi: 10.1126/science.1125949.

Weissleder, R. & Ntziachristos, V. (2003). "Shedding light onto live molecular targets." *Nature medicine, 9*, 123. doi:10.1038/nm0103-123.

Weissleder, R., Bogdanov, A., Neuwelt, E. A. & Papisov, M. (1995). "Long-circulating iron oxides for MR imaging." *Advanced Drug Delivery Reviews, 16*, 321-334. doi:10.1016/0169-409x(95)00033-4.

Weller, H. (1993). "Colloidal semiconductor q-particles: chemistry in the transition region between solid state and molecules." *Angewandte*

Chemie International Edition in English, *32*, 41-53. doi:10.1002/anie.199300411.

Weller, H. (1998). "Quantum size colloids: From size-dependent properties of discrete particles to self-organized superstructures." *Current opinion in colloid & interface science*, *3*, 194-199. doi:10.1016/s1359-0294(98)80013-7

Weller, H. (1993). "A novel state of matter for materials science." *Adv. Mater*, *5*, 88-95. doi: 10.1002/adma.19930050204.

Wirtz, C. R., Knauth, M., Staubert, A., Bonsanto, M. M., Sartor, K., Kunze, S. & Tronnier, V. M. (2000). "Clinical evaluation and follow-up results for intraoperative magnetic resonance imaging in neurosurgery." *Neurosurgery*, *46*, 1112-1122. doi:10.1097/00006123-200005000-00017.

Woods, M., Botta, M., Avedano, S., Wang, J. & Sherry, A. D. (2005). "Towards the rational design of MRI contrast agents: a practical approach to the synthesis of gadolinium complexes that exhibit optimal water exchange. *Dalton Transactions*, *24*, 3829-3837. doi:10.1039/b510778d.

Yanushevich, Y. G., Shagin, D. A., Fradkov, A. F., Shakhbazov, K. S., Barsova, E. V., Gurskaya, N. G. & Lukyanov, S. A. (2005). "Spectral diversity among members of the green fluorescent protein family in hydroid jellyfish (Cnidaria, Hydrozoa)." *Russian Journal of Bioorganic Chemistry*, *31*, 43-47.doi:10.1007/s11171-005-0005-9.

Ye, Y., Bloch, S., Kao, J. & Achilefu, S. (2005). "Multivalent carbocyanine molecular probes: synthesis and applications." *Bioconjugate chemistry*, *16*, 51-61. doi:10.1021/ bc049790i.

Yin, J., Hu, Y. & Yoon, J. (2015). "Fluorescent probes and bioimaging: alkali metals, alkaline earth metals and pH." *Chemical Society Reviews*, *44*, 4619-4644. doi:10.1039/c4cs00275j.

Yoon, T. J., Yu, K. N., Kim, E., Kim, J. S., Kim, B. G., Yun, S. H. & Park, S. B. (2006). "Specific targeting, cell sorting, and bioimaging with smart magnetic silica core–shell nanomaterials. *Small*, *2*, 209-215. doi:10.1002/smll.200500360.

Zeng, S., Tsang, M. K., Chan, C. F., Wong, K. L. & Hao, J. (2012). "PEG modified BaGdF5: Yb/Ernanoprobes for multi-modal upconversion fluorescent, *in vivo* X-ray computed tomography and biomagnetic imaging." *Biomaterials*, *33*, 9232-9238. doi: 10.1016/ j.biomaterials. 2012.09.019.

Zhao, H., Doyle, T. C., Coquoz, O., Kalish, F., Rice, B. W. & Contag, C. H. (2005). "Emission spectra of bioluminescent reporters and interaction with mammalian tissue determine the sensitivity of detection *in vivo*." *Journal of biomedical optics*, *10*, 041210. doi:10.1117/1.2032388.

Zhao, Y., Pang, B., Luehmann, H., Detering, L., Yang, X., Sultan, D. & Liu, Y. (2016). "Gold Nanoparticles Doped with 199Au Atoms and Their Use for Targeted Cancer Imaging by SPECT." *Advanced healthcare materials*, *5*, 928-935. doi:10.1002/adhm.201500992.

Zheng, G., Li, H., Yang, K., Blessington, D., Licha, K., Lund-Katz, S. & Glickson, J. D. (2002). "Tricarbocyanine cholesteryl laurates labeled LDL: new near infrared fluorescent probes (NIRFs) for monitoring tumors and gene therapy of familial hypercholesterolemia." *Bioorganic & medicinal chemistry letters*, *12*, 1485-1488. doi: 10.1016/S0960-894X(02)00193-2.

In: Nanoparticles ISBN: 978-1-53616-596-8
Editors: A. K. Samantara, S. Ratha

Chapter 4

NANOMATERIALS IN TISSUE ENGINEERING AND MRI APPLICATION

Swarnabala Jena*
College of Basic Science and Humanities,
Odisha University of Agriculture and Technology,
Bhubaneswar, Odisha, India

ABSTRACT

Tissue engineering (TE) is an advanced technology which cultivates substitutes for damaged tissues in the living body. It develops engineered methods for material production, cell combination and growth factors. Tissue engineering uses scaffolds to form new tissues which are then implemented in medical therapy. Hence, it is also called as regenerative medicine. The whole body information is detected by different imaging methods used in tissue engineering. Among them, Magnetic Resonance Imaging (MRI) is considered as an excellent imaging technique, because of its high resolution and applicability in both in vitro and in vivo studies. It uses strong magnetic field and radio-waves for imaging, which produces a detailed image of cell death, inflammation, cell division, cell

* Corresponding Author's Email: swarnajena.chem@gmail.com.

transformation, cell growth and gene expression, inside the body. It also visualizes the images of tissue implant and its surroundings thereafter. The scaffold used in TE is a three dimensional porous structure which is biocompatible with the cells. These scaffolds are treated as supports for tissue growth, which commands cells to grow into correct anatomical shape. There are various substrates that have been used for the purpose of tissue growth, and recently, nanomaterials, especially carbon nanotubes have been reported to be used as suitable scaffold for tissue growth due to their attracting tubular size and surface area along with exciting physicochemical properties. This chapter briefly describes the details of TE, different imaging modalities, especially MRI and its application, use of nanomaterials in TE and MRI application.

Keywords: tissue engineering, nanoparticles, MRI, composites

1. Tissue Engineering

Tissue engineering, which forms an important component of "regenerative medicine," is of interest, as it generates new biological cells or tissues for impaired tissues in living organisms. It replaces, restores and regenerates cells by obeying certain engineering principles. The application of tissue engineering covers approximately all the fields of science, especially in medicinal therapy. According to Langer and Vacanti, tissue engineering is an interdisciplinary field, which applies to the principles of both engineering and life science, and produces biological substitutes which restore, maintain and improve biological tissue function (Langer et al. 1993, 920). Presently, transplant, surgery and mechanical devices are used as tissue damage therapy. But, the hurdles associated with these therapies are, lack of suitable donor for transplant, inadequate transplantation, long term post-surgery problems, and incapability of mechanical device to accomplish all the tissue functions (Castells et al. 2013, 004). Tissue engineering is applied both in vitro and in vivo culture of cells and tissues. Hence, it is a promising technique for tissue engineers for various applications. Tissue engineering combines cells, provides scaffolds for tissue growth, assimilates growth factors. Generally, natural or synthetic materials are used as scaffold for substitute tissues, which have excellent biocompatibility. The scaffolds are made from collagen or decomposable polymers. Substitute tissues are formed by planting human cells into the scaffolds, which holds growth factors for cell division and trigger the regenerative process. The growth factors direct cells in the scaffolds to form exact anatomical shape of the tissues that are to be substituted. The prepared tissue can be set into the human body along with the implanted scaffold, which finally get absorbed or dissolved inside the body. Normally, skin, cartilage, heart, and bone related damages can be prevented and treated by tissue engineering. The source for cell construction is human embryonic stem cells which are cultured in vitro. Embryonic stem cells are differentiated into many tissues, i.e., mesenchymal stem cells, which can be separated into fat, bone, cartilage, muscle, ligament, tendon, and marrow stroma. The in vitro cultured stem cells produce cells for tissue replacement and regeneration and used in therapy of varieties of diseases related to skin, bone, liver, cardiac, neurological and brain. For a particular type of therapy in humans, the embryonic stem cells are first selected, then engineered for cell production, growth and separation and grafting. Figure 1 shows a general method of TE applied as regenerative medicine.

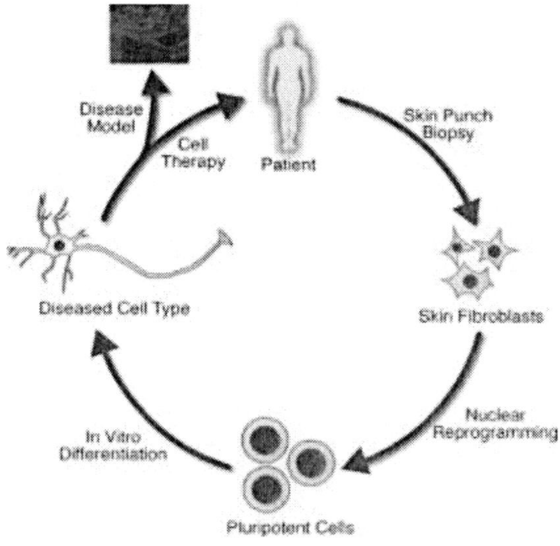

Figure 1. An overview of TE as regenerative medicine.

2. IMAGING IN TISSUE ENGINEERING

Tissue engineering, its varied research and related innovative tools are used in various arenas of science and it has motivated research towards in vitro, and mostly medical therapy applications. In tissue engineering, tissue engineers make use of a 3D porous scaffold which contains cells, growth factors and biomolecules for tissue growth. This is possible only if tissue engineers have a distinct picture of cell, extracellular matrix and biological growth factors (Huihui et al. 2008, 515). There are several imaging methods of TE, which displays morphological, functional and molecular levels of information inside the body. Previously, several conventional techniques, i.e., histological techniques, have been used to get information regarding in vivo cultured transplants, before and after applications. But, this information is very limited for longitudinal three-dimensional (3D) volumetric assessments (Appel et al. 2013, 6615). Hence, the modern imaging techniques overcome the limitations of the previously used conventional methods. A perfect imaging technology gives signals of high resolution, enters deep through the whole body and displays all the basic information regarding morphological, physiological, and molecular changes at subcellular level. For various applications in tissue engineered constructs, one single imaging modality is not sufficient to give all the information. Every imaging method has special applications. They provide information in a particular range and it depends upon the properties of the imaging system. Various imaging modalities used now–a-days are as per the requirement of tissue engineering constructs. Generally, the imaging methods, which are used for various TE applications are, X-ray and computed tomography (CT), positron emission tomography (PET), single photon emission computed tomography (SPECT), magnetic resonance imaging (MRI), ultrasound imaging, optical imaging, and multimodal imaging (Nam et al. 2014).

2.1. X-Ray and CT Imaging

X-ray and CT are two important diagnostic techniques for bone tissue injury and fracture. The images obtained through these techniques have excellent spatial resolutions (Brenner and Hall 2007, 2277; Fleischmann and Boas 2011, 510). The energy source for these imaging methods is X-ray and this energy enters the cores of the human body to create the image. The tissue absorbs photons from an X-ray beam in relation to the electron density of the tissue. The number of photons passing through the injury site detects images through the decrease in the intensity of the applied X-ray beam. The resulting images are a two-dimensional projection of a three-dimensional structure (Johansson 2015, 189). The electromagnetic radiations used for imaging purpose have very high energy signatures as compared to the electromagnetic energy found in the case of visible spectra. Due to their high electromagnetic energy, X-ray source in X-ray imaging and CT has deep penetration depth and outstanding sensitivity and is used to determine the structure of bone and other diagnostic applications. But, some limitations of such high energy X-ray beam is that it can structurally modify and/or destructs soft tissue or the samples which are under test. Still, it is a powerful tool for bone imaging. The bone structures after healing, its morphological changes, and the in vivo and ex vivo study of bone growth and its connection to scaffolds are also checked through CT and X-ray imaging. The properties of tissue-engineered constructs, i.e., sponginess, pore size, and internal connections of tissues or bones with adjacent or other tissues are also measured by using both X-ray and CT imaging techniques (Papantoniou et al. 2014, 177; Giuliani et al. 2014, 308). CT imaging is enhanced by contrast agents. Hexabrix is generally used as a CT imaging contrast agent, which is coated onto the scaffolds to enhance the nano-CT imaging. In vitro cultured silk fibroin frameworks with chondrocytes are imaged by Hexabrix-enriched micro-CT. These images give information regarding proteoglycan production and maximum scaffold production conditions for cartilage tissue engineering (Wang et al. 2010, 4672). But, the limitation with the contrast agents is that much of the imaging data is lost during the test. X-ray phase-contrast micro-CT imaging is superior to contrast agents as contrast agents are lethal and need fixing of tasters. Generally, traditional X-ray imaging cannot image soft tissues properly, due to low contrast. But, phase contrast X-ray imaging can easily measure the images of these soft tissues and are sensitive. Hence, CT and X-ray imaging also gives information about structural and morphological changes of tissue-engineered builds. Cells, cell distribution on 3D scaffold, cell movement in vivo, are examined by X-ray imaging. Cells are labelled with either iron oxide or gold nanoparticles to enhance the contrast for imaging (Thimm et al. 2011, 167; Farini et al. 2012, 3059).

2.2. Magnetic Resonance Imaging (MRI)

MRI is a whole body medical diagnostic technique that possesses exceptional imaging transmission, high penetration depth, and operational safety, and also is applicable to both in vitro and in vivo studies. In this technique, atoms are placed in a strong magnetic field of 1.5–10 T and the nuclei, i.e., ^{1}H in the body is allied in the direction of the field. The magnetic moment spins round the atom at the Larmor frequency. Radio frequency pulse used, determines the extent of magnetization and the frequency. As per the pulse command, longitudinal or transversal magnetization relaxation times (T1 or T2) and proton density are identified and shown as MR image. Micro-MRI is useful for tissue engineers for three-dimensional resolution (*100 μm) at higher magnetic fields of strength 7–9 T (Nam et al. 2014). The structural, functional and cellular information are measured by MRI and it can be achieved by using various contrast agents such as gadolinium- or iron oxide and magnetic nanoparticles (Jun et al. 2008, 5122; Terreno et al. 2010, 3019). MRI can measure cell decay, inflammation, cell transformation and gene expression. When a tissue is grafted completely, then the mixing of tissue with the neighbouring tissues and the quick signs of immune rejection are measured by using MRI. In vitro studies such as assessment of the composition of bladder a cellular matrix based scaffolds are measured by MRI using MR relaxation times (T1, T2) and diffusion coefficients (Cheng et al. 2010,

341). MRI is used to assess the intermediate adhesive layers after the incorporation of hydrogel in cartilage (Ramaswamy et al. 2006, 144).

2.3. Ultrasound Imaging

Ultrasound imaging is an analytical method for diagnosis of small sized samples. It is biocompatible, exhibits high chronological resolution, sensitive, transferable, cost effective, and has high perception depth (Ntziachristos 2010, 603). Ultrasound waves are transmitted and received by a single or an array of transducer, by reflection and backscattering. The penetration depth and resolution of ultrasound imaging are scalable, and used for various applications. The acoustic impedance difference between the density and bulk moduli of the medium gives ultrasound images. Hence, ultrasound imaging gives mechanical and morphological data of tissue-engineered constructs both for in vitro and in vivo testing conditions (Nam et al. 2014, 115). The collagen content of fibrin-based tissue-engineered structures and mineralization in collagen hydrogels are quantitatively analysed by ultrasound scans (Kreitz et al. 2011, 1021; Gudur et al. 2012, 935). The mechanical properties and their localization in the sections of tissue-engineered cartilage after transplantation of the constructs in the subcutaneous areas of nude mice for 2 months is examined by using high frequency ultrasound microscopy (Tanaka et al. 2012, 252). The quantitative measurement of mechanical properties of soft tissues are not measured by the conventional ultrasound imaging. Ultrasound elastography is useful for this purpose (Garra 2007, 255; Wells et al. 2011, 1521; Bercoff et al. 2004, 396; Deffieux et al. 2009, 313). The surface irregularity, morphology change and nonlinear elastic properties of engineered oral mucosal tissues in ex vivo are monitored by ultrasound elastography (Winterroth 2011, 1734; Winterroth 2012, 345; Abraham 2000, 956). The mechanical property changes in biodegradable polyurethane scaffolds implanted in the rat muscular abdominal wall in vivo is monitored by ultrasound elasticity imaging (Yu et al. 2013, 2701).

3. Nanostructures in Tissue Engineering

Tissue engineering has wide application in numerous fields of science. By applying various innovative in vivo and in vitro cultured methods, it provides biological substitutes which are useful to regenerate, replace, and retain the ill tissues in the body. The TE constructs also increases the cell, tissue and organ functions. In short, we call TE as an efficient technology which incorporates all branches of science, i.e., engineering, biological, medicinal, material and chemical. Generally, TE techniques which are used till now, face various shortcomings which include presence of insufficient compatible biomaterials, lack of appropriate tissue scaffold for tissue development, unproductive cell growth, formation of inefficient growth factors and its fruitless direction for tissue growth in cell and incapability to control cell functions and properties. Nanoparticles overcome these limitations of TE application and constructs due to its small size and high surface to volume ratio. The Nanoscale ranges of nanoparticles and their physicochemical properties encourage tissue engineers to implement TE in wide range of applications. Hence, these are used in TE to enhance the mechanical, biological, physiochemical properties of tissue engineered constructs. In medical research, nanoparticles are used for drug delivery, bio sensing, DNA construction, gene delivery, localising specific ill site (Wilson et al. 2010, 923; Shi et al. 210, 3223; Mironov et al. 2008, 338; Koo 2005, 193; Furno et al. 2004, 1019). Some of the examples of nanoparticles, which are used recently are, gold nanoparticles (GNPs), silver and other nanoparticles, metal oxide nanoparticles, quantum dots etc. GNPs have high electrical conductivity and its surface conjugation with other tissues make them an interesting material for TE constructs. Metallic nanoparticles like silver and some other metals and metal oxides possess antimicrobial properties which enables them for various TE applications. Recently, quantum dots have been used in imaging techniques due to their fluorescence properties. Another most widely used nanomaterial is carbon nanotubes (CNTs), which has excellent electrochemical properties that can be exploited in numerous TE applications. Magnetic nanoparticles (MNPs) are exciting material for tissue engineers used for cell mechanotransduction, gene delivery, cell designing and construction of 3D tissue scaffolds. The size of nanoparticles is generally compared with the size of proteins and peptides so they diffuse through the membranes and penetrate inside the cells. They mimic extracellular matrix (ECM) components of tissues (Anwarul et al. 2018, 5637–5655). Due to their nanosize, nanomaterials are used as starting materials for molecular structure construction and act as a bridge between the macro and microscopic structures. They show slow sedimentation rates due to high mobility in their free state. Nanomaterials exhibit quantum effect which enables them to take control over initial protein adsorption to dictate cellular interactions (Khang et al. 2007, 4756). These properties make nanoparticles potential candidates to be used in biomedical, optoelectronics, and many more interesting applications.

3.1. Carbon Nanostructures for Tissue Engineering Scaffolds

In tissue engineering, the tissue growth is supported by a three dimensional porous structure called scaffold. The main function of scaffold in tissue engineering is to provide necessary spatial composition to cells for tissue growth and to hint the cells to form exact anatomical shape. A tissue engineering scaffold must be biocompatible to the cells that are to be grown, avoid cell inhibition, and have the ability to transport nutrients and wastes. Nanostructure developed tissue engineering scaffolds have different functions and the function depends on their size and shape. The properties of nanomaterials also design the scaffolds. For instance, neural tissue requires nano scaffolds having electrical conductivity, while bone and cartilage cells require mechanical properties based scaffolds. These scaffolds are prepared from nanomaterials at the required nanoscale sizes. The properties of nanostructures depend on the nanomaterial used. Now-a-days, carbon nanotube is used in tissue engineering due to their excellent electrical conductivity, chemical and mechanical stability, rigidity, and have the potential to be used as scaffolds. Extracellular matrix present in the cell supports the surrounding cells to grow efficiently and increases cell functions. Filamentous carbon nanotubes possess the same structural composition as extracellular matrix and facilitates the cell growth. Hence, carbon nanotubes have the ability to increase the cell function as the extracellular matrix in the cell (Tran et al. 2009, 1097). Cells, which are linked directly onto the carbon nanotube surface are biocompatible with it and produce excellent cell growth. For example, in bone, neural and cardiac tissue engineering carbon nanotubes prove as best tissue engineered scaffold. Osteoblasts, osteoclasts and osteocytes are the cells formed in bone tissue engineering. Previously used nanomaterials for bone tissue engineering lacked desired mechanical strength. But, it has been found by various studies that carbon nanotubes show highest strength for bone tissue engineering and is compatible with bone cells. Multi-walled carbon nanotubes have been used for bone repairing and are successfully integrated into new bone. In the future, bone tissue engineering would be useful to support artificial bone implants and could be applied in hard tissue surgery. Nanotubes are used in neural tissue engineering, because its tubular structure mimics the natural tubular forms and can produce micro-tubes. Carbon nanotubes possess high electrical conductivity and may be used to maintain electrical signals between neuronal cells. Studies have found that neuronal cells can grow euritis onto carbon nanotube substrates and by changing the orientation of the carbon nanotubes, the direction of neurite growth can be controlled. Due to electrical conducting property of carbon nanotubes, it is used in cardiac tissue engineering. The cardiovascular defects and heart failure in the body are cured by regenerating cardiac tissue. Carbon nanotubes are used to develop devices which are implanted in damaged tissue for functioning cardiac tissues. A 2D patch is formed by embedding carbon nanotubes into gelatin methacrylate hydrogels, which is used for the engineering of cardiomyocytes and the cells produced showed synchronous beating. Carbon nanotubes used for this engineering act as agent to enhances cell-cell adhesion and cell-cell electrical coupling (Nanotechnology in Tissue Engineering. WWW.azonano.com, 2017).

3.2. Application of Nanoparticles in Tissue Engineering

Due to their unique physical, chemical, mechanical, biological and electrical properties, nanoparticles have varied application in various fields. In TE, nanoparticles are used in gene delivery, DNA transfection, viral transduction, cell patterning, and bio sensing (Anwarul et al. 2018, 5637–5655). Depending on their size, shape and structure, nanoparticles are used in TE to enhance the biological, mechanical and electrical properties of scaffolds and its function. Generally, nanoparticles of size 1-100 nm determine the properties of bulk material and molecular structure (Anwarul et al. 2018, 5637–5655; Radomska et al. 2016, 151). The properties and applications, which are enhanced by nanoparticles in TE are given below.

3.2.1. Biological Property

Depending on their size and intrinsic property and biocompatibility with the cells nanoparticles are used to increase the cell performance, cell production and tissue engineering scaffold. Typically GNPs and titanium dioxide (TiO_2) nanoparticles are used to enhance cell proliferation rates in bone and cardiac tissue regeneration (Anwarul et al. 2018, 5637–5655). Previously, bone morphogenetic proteins (BMPs) were being used in bone tissue regeneration and repairing (Bessa et al. 2008, 81; Lim et al. 2014, 7). But, the shortcomings such as high cost, susceptibility towards unwanted bone formation, inflammation reactions were greater than the benefits. GNPs overcome these limitations of BMPs and have effectively replaced them in bone tissue engineering, as the former is biocompatible and can modify the surface of the cells, efficiently. Some of the important application of GNPs in bone tissue engineering has been discussed here, which are the reports obtained by several researchers. For example, promotion of osteogenic differentiation of an osteoblast precursor cell MC3T3-E1, osteoclast formation in hematopoietic cells, prevention of mitochondrial dysfunction in osteoblastic cells, osteogenic and adipogenic differentiation in mesenchymal stem cells (MSCs), during the p38 mitogen-activated protein kinase (MAPK) pathway are promoted by GNPs

(Boisselier and Astruc 2009, 1759; Chen et al. 2015, 8938; Ko 2015, 68; Suh et al. 2013, 428). The size of GNPs also influences the osteogenic differentiation, e.g., 30–50 nm GNPs are effective for human adipose-derived stem cell (ADSC) function, while 20-40 nm sized GNPs are useful for MC3T3-E1 osteoblast cell function (Ko 2015, 68; Liu et al. 2010, 1013). Hybrid scaffolds, i.e., GNPs and gelatin are effective for osteogenic differentiation of humans' adipose stem cells (Heo et al. 2014, 1584). GNPs and gold nanowire scaffold have been used in cell proliferation, synapse formation and stem cell differentiation without using growth factors (Subbiah et al. 2010, 4559; Jaconi 2011, 692). GNP-loaded nanofibers enhance cardiomyogenic cells differentiation leading to infarcted myocardium regeneration (Ravichandran 2014, 515). TiO_2 nanoparticles with human embryonic stem cell derived cardiomyocytes scaffolds have reportedly shown enhanced cell proliferation (Jawad et al. 2008, 31). Furthermore, TiO_2 nanoparticles with poly (lactic-co-glycolic acid) (PLGA) have been used to improve bone cell performance (Liu et al. 2006, 541). The dangerous effects of acid by-products released by PLGA during degradation are minimized by TiO_2 nanoparticles (Wanjale et al. 2006, 6414).

3.2.2. Mechanical Property

Nanocomposite polymers in hydrogels and electrospun fibers show outstanding mechanical property for TE applications (El Fray et al. 2005, 2300; Liu et al. 2008, 1005; Jawad et al. 2011, 372). TiO_2-embedded scaffold shows high tensile strength for myocardial infarction (Lim et al. 2015, 1606). Hydrogel microfibers in poly (N-isopropylacrylamide) and MNPs increase the mechanical properties of hydrogel microfibers (Wang et al. 2016, 1228). Attapulgite nanoparticles increase the mechanical properties of chitosan/β-glycerophosphate disodium salt (CS/GP). The hydrogen bonds formed between attapulgite nanoparticles and CS molecules show fivefold larger tensile strength and elongation as compared to CS/GP hydrogel (Wang et al. 2016, 1228). A mixture of type I collagen and polyvinylpyrrolidone (PVP)-coated TiO_2 nanoparticles have been used for skin TE application. The hydrogen bonds formed between collagen,

PVP and TiO_2; improve the tensile strength of the scaffolds (Kubota et al. 1994, 1107; Li et al. 2016, 287). GNPs, silver nanoparticles and MNPs embedded scaffolds improve the scaffold mechanics, and hydroxyapatite (HA) nanoparticles enhance the mechanical properties of electro spun silk fibroin scaffolds (Luderer et al. 2013, 219; Kim et al. 2014, 324). CNTs, owing to their notable mechanical properties, tensile strength and fiber-like structure, are used in TE applications and can readily enhance the properties of polymers (Gonçalves et al. 2016, 1210; Ju et al. 2008, 136; Han et al. 2013, 11058). CNTs enforced polylactic acid (PLA) blends, electrospun into nanofiber mats shows superior osteoinductive potential than PLA/gelatin nanofibers (Magiera et al. 2017, 11). CNTs, with polycaprolactone (PCL), increase the mechanical properties of PCL and enhance the proliferation and differentiation of rat bone marrow stem cells (BMSCs) (Pan et al. 2012, 226). Graphene oxide (GO) and silk fibroin composite improves proliferation, adhesion and viability of human periodontal ligament mesenchymal stem cells (PDLSCs) (Rodríguez-Lozano et al. 2015, 399). Graphene-based nanomaterials of stem cells increase the mechanical properties along with enhanced proliferation, attachment, osteogenic differentiation, and bone regeneration (Feng et al. 2011, 317; Kim et al. 2013, 933; Chen et al. 2012, 418).

3.2.3. Electrical Property

Nanoparticles enhance the electrical properties of scaffolds and are used in cardiac TE (Ravichandran et al. 2014, 515). Myocardial infarction is treated with GNPs deposited over fibrous decellularized matrices scaffolds (Shevach et al. 2014, 5792). Gold nanostructures-integrated scaffolds increase matrix conductivity and develop electrical signal between different cardiac components. GNP-based electrospun fibrous scaffold is used for cardiac tissue regeneration. The infarcted heart function is improved by the nanocomposites prepared from GNPs deposited gelatin and PCL–gelatin fibers (Shevach et al. 2013, 5210; Navaei et al. 2016, 133; Kharaziha et al. 2016, 1533). Gold nanowires, along with the scaffolds, are used to enhance the electrical conductivity of cells and synapse formation of cardiac muscle cells (Shin et al. 2015,

4486). CNTs with polymer composites improve electrical conductivity and promote cardiomyocyte functions (Stout et al. 2011, 3101). Table-1 shows the electrical conductivity of nanocomposites and their application (Anwarul et al. 2018, 5637–5655).

Table 1. Electrical conductivity of nanocomposites and their applications in the biomedical field. Obtained with permission from Anwarul et al. 2018, 5637–5655

Polymer	Polymers' conductivity (S cm^{-1}), before adding nanoparticles	Nanocomposites	Nanocomposites' conductivity (S cm^{-1}), after adding nanoparticles	Applications
Chitosan	7.4×10^{-9}	Chitosan/carbon	3.08×10^{-3}	Cardiac TE
PANI	10^{-3}	PANI/Ag	10^{-2}	TE and wound-healing applications
Hydrogel	0.23±0.02	Graphene/hydrogel	4.9±0.2	TE applications
PPy	1.3×10^{-5}	PPy/chitosan	10^{-3}–10^{-7}	TE and wound-healing applications
PPy	1.3×10^{-5}	PPy/cellulose acetate	6.9×10^{-4} to 3.6×10^{1}	TE applications
PANI	10^{-3}	PANI nanofibers/collagen	0.27	Scaffold material for biomedical applications
PANI	10^{-3}	PANI nanofiber/bacterial cellulose	10^{-2}	Biosensors, TE
PPy	1.3×10^{-5}	PPy nanoparticles/PU	2.3×10^{-6}	TE
PPy	1.3×10^{-5}	PPy/poly(d,l-lactic acid)	15.65×10^{-3}	Synthetic nerve conduits
PU	8.8×10^{-11}	PU/graphene	$.10^{-3}$	Sensors, bone applications
PMMA	10^{-11}	PMMA/MwCNT	10^{-5}	Devices for TE

Abbreviations: TE, tissue engineering; PANI, polyaniline; PPy, polypyrrole; PU, polyurethane; PMMA, polymethylmethacrylate; MwCNT, multiwalled carbon nanotubes.

3.2.4. Gene Delivery

Gene delivery utilizes human mesenchymal stem cells (hMSCs) in TE. These cells are immunesuppressive, and differentiate into chondrocytes, osteoblasts, myocytes and adipocytes (Pittenger et al. 1999, 143; Wang et al. 2012, 23357). Gene delivery system should possess high gene transfection efficiency, low cytotoxicity and high specificity to unhealthy cells. The nanomaterials play a vital role for both the processes in gene delivery. Gene delivery is of two types: viral and nonviral. Non-viral methods are simple and secure and are used for DNA transfection (Ito and Kamihira 2011, 355). Magnetofection is used in gene delivery for DNA transfection which uses MNPs. In this technique, the plasmid DNA, cationic lipids, polymer complexes of DNA, first interact with the magnetic beads. Then the magnetic force attracts them towards the target cells and accumulates on the surface (Scherer et al. 2002, 102). Methods of magnetofection are also associated with Lipofectamine, polyethyleneimine or dioleoyltrimethylammounium for gene delivery (Scherer et al. 2002, 102). In endothelial cells and embryonic stem cells, magnetofection also shows high expression levels in target cells (Krötz et al. 2003, 425; Lee et al. 2008, 133). Fibroblasts and keratinocytes, by using reporter genes, show transfection efficiencies, which are respectively, 36- and 10-fold higher than the cationic liposomes (Ino et al. 2008, 168). Iron oxide magnetic particles, CNTs and nickel embedded magnetic nanotubes are also used as efficient gene delivery agents for DNA transfection (Neuberger et al. 2005, 483; Haris et al. 2003, 1367; Khan et al. 2011, 1947; Alshehri et al. 2016, 8149; Cai et al. 2005, 449). In viral transduction, viral vectors with titer are developed and applied in TE. Retroviral vectors are captured by magnetite cationic liposomes (MCLs) and seeded into mouse neuroblastoma cells and the viral titer is increased by 55-fold (Ito et al. 2008, 57). The physical interactions due to magnetic force increase the cellular uptakes of magnetic nanoparticles (Anwarul et al. 2018, 5637–5655).

3.3. Application of Nanoparticles IN MRI

Recent technology demands new techniques for a non-invasive assessment of tissues inside the human body. Early diagnosis and imaging methods are incorporated with the new techniques and used in medical therapy. Among the various imaging modality, MRI is successful due to its high spatial resolution, non-invasive and non-destructive nature (Mankoff 2007, 18N). The MR images can be visualized by measuring the relaxation times, both longitudinally (T1) and transversally (T2). But, the technological hurdle for the determination of any diseases by MRI is that it gives the same intense signal in the case of both the target cells and the surrounding healthy cells as well (Yadollahpour et al. 2017). Hence, the use of contrast agents (CAs) drastically enhance the imaging ability. Contrast agents change the proton T1 and T2 relaxation time by interacting with water molecules (Shellock and Kanal 1999, 477; Caravan et al. 2009, 89). Recently, nanoparticles have been reported to play a paramount role and act as CAs in MRI due to their high magnetization value, small size and effectiveness in both in vivo and in vitro applications (Yadollahpour et al. 2017; Ali et al. 2015, 131; Yadollahpour 2015, 271; Yadollahpour and Rashidi 2015, 25). Commonly used NPs are iron oxide, gold and gadolinium etc. Paramagnetic NPs are used as T1 CAs while super paramagnetic NPs are termed as T2 CAs. Gadolinium is used as T1 CAs in MRI but its toxicity causes renal failure in patients. Hence, iron oxide can be a potential alternative, but it has a characteristic relaxivity issue (Yadollahpour et al. 2017, S7). SPIONs are the contrast agent in MRI, for determining cellular and molecular level images (Bulte and Kraitchman 2004, 484; Smirnov et al. 2006, 498; Billotey et al. 2005, 579; Hao et al. 2010, 2729; Yadollahpour et al. 2016, 11451; Yadollahpour et al. 2016, 14737; Yadollahpour and Venkateshwarlu 2016, 11379). Size of nanoparticles also influences the imaging process. SPIONs are the iron oxide NPs having diameter between 1-100 nm, and they are generally found in the form of magnetite and maghemite. Magnetite has an inverse spinel structure with oxygen and form fcc lattice in which tetrahedral sites are occupied by the Fe^{3+} species and octahedral sites are occupied by both Fe^{2+} and Fe^{3+} ions. In maghemite, iron is found in a +3 oxidation state and cation vacancies in octahedral site form a cubic unit cell (Bulte and Kraitchman 2004, 484; Yadollahpour et al. 2017, S7; Laurent et al. 2008, 2064; Andreas et al. 2012, 4515; Cha et al. 2011, 152; Hu et al. 2011, 245604; Yang et al. 2011, 4584). Gadolinium nanoparticles are regarded as efficient relaxation enhancing agents due to the presence of seven unpaired electrons (Brasch 1983, 781; Brasch 2005, 423). The five electrons catalyse the relaxation rate of water hydrogen atoms producing positive contrast (Caravan et al. 1999, 2293). Gadolinium oxides with size less than 65 nm show relaxivity, which is less than 20/s/Mm (Yadollahpour et al. 2017, S7). Though Gd^{3+} is a good contrast agent in MRI application, it is very toxic and interferes with the calcium channel and protein binding sites (Yadollahpour and Venkateshwarlu 2016, 11379; Lansman 1990, 679; Biagi and Enyeart 1990, C515; Faucher et al. 2012, 4506; Xu et al. 2012, 10907; Zhang et al. 2012, 14494; Zhang et al. 2014, 356). The toxic effects of Gd^{3+} ions are reduced by combining it with chelating ligands (Yadollahpour et al. 2017, S7). Au NPs of size less than 13 nm are good CAs in MRI due to their high surface modification capacity (Alric et al. 2008, 5908; Park et al. 2010, 2287; Chen et al. 2013, 5200; Wen et al. 2013, 1570). Yadollahpour et al. (2017, S7) give a detailed review of different CAs used in MRI which has been shown in a Table 2.

CONCLUSION

Advancement of new technology in TE and MRI is beneficial for clinical therapy. Nanoparticles, due to their unique properties have advantages over others and have successfully been used for both TE and MRI applications due to their biocompatibility, size, shape and surface area. Various nanoparticles are used as TE scaffolds for therapeutic treatments, which act as support structures for tissue growth. The nanomaterial-embedded TE scaffolds direct cells to grow and form exact anatomical shapes. For the detection of diseases, nanomaterials can be used as CAs in MRI technique. The detection also depends upon the size of nanoparticles. Various nanoparticles, used for both TE and MRI, are toxic, e.g., gadolinium, iron oxides. Recently used paramagnetic and super paramagnetic nanoparticles have been found to be even more beneficial over them.

Table 2. Characteristics of the reviewed studies. Obtained with permission from Yadollahpour et al. 2017, S7

Study	**Contrast agent**	**Size**	**Test**	**Disease**	**Dose**	**Relaxivity (mM/S)**	**Outcome**
Xie et al., 2011; China	Lf-SPIONs	75 nm	In vivo (animal)	Brain gliomas	51 emu/g Fe	r2=75.6	Enhanced T2W after 48 h
Xie et al., 2011; China	Fe_3O_4 at SiO_2	21 nm	In vitro and in vivo (animal)	Glio-blastoma tumors	200 mL (2 mg/mL)	r1=4.2 r2=17.4	Extended for fabricating other biologically active NPs
Im et al., 2012; Korea	Fe_3O_4/MnO hybrid	5, 11, and 21 nm	In vitro and in vivo (animal)	HCC	20 ml	r1 remained unaffected, r2 78.9 and 141	Detection of HCC with a high degree of conspicuity
Cha et al., 2011; Korea	PCM-CS	43.1±6.3 nm	In vivo (animal)	SCC 7 tumor bearing xeno-grafted	0.05 ml PCM-CS 0.15 mg Fe/mL		NIRF signal of tumor increased up to 12 h post injection
Andreas et al., 2012; Germany	Citrate SPIONs	80-160 nm	In vivo (animal) and ex vivo	MSCs	25 mg Fe/ml citrate, 500 mg Fe/ml Endorem		Very efficient intracellular magnetic labels for in vivo stem cell tracking by MRI
Hu et al., 2011; China	Ultra-small PEGylated iron oxide	5.4 nm	In vitro	HeLa cell		r1=19.7 and the lowest r2/r1 ratio of 2.0	SPIONs have little effect on HeLa cell viability
Chou et al., 2010; Taiwan	FePt	3, 6, and 12 nm	In vitro and in vivo	MBT2 tumor			The 3 nm-FePt showed higher brain concentrations
Lu et al., 2009; China	Mn-SPIO	80 nm	In vitro and in vivo	Hepato carcinoma		r2=270	High sensitive identification of small liver lesions

Study	Contrast agent	Size	Test	Disease	Dose	Relaxivity (mM/S)	Outcome
Zhang et al., 2012; China	GH		In vitro and in vivo	Blood pool and liver	10 mL, 24.2 mM of Gd^{3+}	r1=15.0 r2=19.7	In vivo T1W in living mice shows GH nanoparticles have an intravascular half-life up to 1 h, much longer than that of Gd-DTPA
Zhang et al., 2013; China	Gd-DTPA-FA		In vitro and in vivo	AP			Highly efficient and specific to detect early AP
Xu et al., 2012; South Korea	Fluorescein PEI coated gadolinium oxide (Gd_2O_3)	3.92 and 7.5 nm	In vivo	Liver tumor	0.1 mmol Gd/kg	r1=6.76 r2=20.27	Excellent MRI-CL dual functionality
Liu et al., 2011; China	PLA-PEG-PLL-Gd	69.8±5.3 nm	In vitro and in vivo	HCC	0.6 mM e12.0 mM		Showed great potential in the early diagnosis of liver tumors
Faucher et al. 2012; Canada	Ultra-small PEG-Gd_2O_3	1.3 nm	In vitro and in vivo	Glio-blastoma multiform	0.3-1.1 pg Gd per cell	r1=14.2 r2/r1=1.20	Strong positive contrast enhancement effects in T1W

HCC: Hepatocellular carcinoma, MRI: Magnetic resonance imaging, CT: Computed tomography, SPIONs: Superparamagnetic iron oxide NPs, NPs: anoparticles, AuNP: Gold nanoparticle, PEI: Poly ethylene imine, TEM: Transmission electron microscopy, AP: Acute pancreatitis, MSCs: Mesenchymal stromal cells, SCC: Squamous cell carcinoma, GH: Gadolinium based hybrid, T1W: T1weighted, T2W: T2weighted.

References

Abraham Cohn, N., Kim, B.-S., Erkamp, R.Q., Mooney, D.J., Emelianov, S.Y., Skovoroda, A.R., and O'Donnell, M. 2000. "High-resolution elasticity imaging for tissue engineering." *IEEE Trans Ultrason Ferroelectr Freq Control* 47: 956. doi: 10.1109/58.852079.

Ali Y., Zohre R., Mostafa J., Samaneh R. 2015. "Applications of upconversion nanoparticles in molecular imaging: A review of recent advances and future opportunities." *Biosci Biotechnol Res Asia* 12: 131-140. doi: 10.22377/ajp.v11i01.1083.

Alric C., Taleb J., Le Duc G., Mandon C., Billotey C., Le Meur-Herland A., Brochard T., Vocanson F., Janier M., Perriat P., Roux S., Tillement O. 2008. "Gadolinium chelate coated gold nanoparticles as contrast agents for both X-ray computed tomography and magnetic resonance imaging." *J Am Chem Soc.* 130: 5908-5915. doi: 10.1021/ja078176p.

Alshehri R., Ilyas A. M., Hasan A., Arnaout, A., Ahmed, F., Memic, A. 2016. "Carbon nanotubes in biomedical applications: factors, mechanisms, and remedies of toxicity: miniperspective." *J Med Chem.* 59: 8149–8167. doi: 10.1021/acs.jmedchem.5b01770.

Andreas K., Georgieva R., Ladwig M., Mueller S., Notter M., Sittinger M., Ringe, J. 2012. "Highly efficient magnetic stem cell labeling with citrate-coated superparamagnetic iron oxide nanoparticles for MRI tracking." *Biomaterials* 33: 4515-4525. doi: 10.1016/j.biomaterials. 2012.02.064.

Appel, A. A., Anastasio, M. A., Larson, J. C., and Brey, E. M. 2013. "Imaging challenges in biomaterials and tissue engineering." *Biomaterials* 34: 6615.

Bercoff, J., Tanter, M., and Fink, M. 2004. "Supersonic shear imaging: a new technique for soft tissue elasticity mapping." *IEEE Trans Ultrason Ferroelectr Freq Control* 51: 396. doi: 10.1109/TUFFC. 2004.1295425.

Bessa P. C., Casal M., Reis R. L. 2008. "Bone morphogenetic proteins in tissue engineering: the road from laboratory to clinic, part II (BMP delivery)." *J Tissue Eng Regen Med.* 2: 81–96. doi: 10.1002/term.74.

Biagi B. A., Enyeart J. J. 1990. "Gadolinium blocks low - and high-threshold calcium currents in pituitary cells." *Am J Physiol* 259: C515-520. doi: 10.1152/ajpcell.1990.259.3.C515.

Billotey C., Aspord C., Beuf O., Piaggio E., Gazeau F., Janier M. F., Thivolet, C. 2005. "T-cell homing to the pancreas in autoimmune mouse models of diabetes: In vivo MR imaging." *Radiology* 236: 579-587. doi: 10.1148/radiol.2362040603.

Boisselier E., Astruc D. 2009. "Gold nanoparticles in nanomedicine: preparations, imaging, diagnostics, therapies and toxicity." *Chem Soc Rev.* 38: 1759–1782. doi: 10.1039/B806051G.

Brasch R. C. 1983. "Work in progress: Methods of contrast enhancement for NMR imaging and potential applications." *A subject review. Radiology* 147: 781-788. doi: 10.1148/radiology.147.3.6342034.

Brasch R. C. 2005. "Contrast-Enhanced NMR Imaging: Animal Studies Using Gadolinium-DTPA Complex." *Classic Papers in Modern Diagnostic Radiology* 423.

Brenner, D. J., and Hall, E. J. 2007. "Computed tomography—an increasing source of radiation exposure." *N Engl J Med* 357: 2277. doi: 10.1056/NEJMra072149.

Bulte J. W., Kraitchman D. L. 2004. "Iron oxide MR contrast agents for molecular and cellular imaging." *NMR Biomed.* 17: 484-99. doi: 10.1002/nbm.924.

Cai D., Mataraza J. M., Qin Z. H., Huang, Z., Huang, J., Chiles, T. C., Carnahan, D., Kempa K., Ren, Z. 2005. "Highly efficient molecular delivery into mammalian cells using carbon nanotube spearing." *Nat Methods.* 2: 449–454. doi: 10.1038/nmeth761.

Caravan P., Ellison J. J., McMurry T. J., Lauffer R. B. 1999. "Gadolinium(III) chelates as MRI contrast agents: Structure, dynamics, and applications." *Chem Rev.* 99: 2293-2352. doi: 10.1021/cr980440x.

Caravan P., Farrar C. T., Frullano L., Uppal R. 2009. "Influence of molecular parameters and increasing magnetic field strength on relaxivity of gadolinium and manganesebased T1 contrast agents." *Contrast Media Mol Imaging* 4: 89-100. doi: 10.1002/cmmi.267.

Castells S. C., Alemany R. M., Fernandez M. T., Recha S. L, Lopez C. P. 2013. "Current Applications of Tissue Engineering in Biomedicine." *J Biochip Tissue chip* S2:004. doi:10.4172/2153-0777.S2-004.

Cha E. J., Jang E. S., Sun I. C., Lee I. J., Ko J. H., Kim Y. I., Kwon, I. C., Kim, K., Ahn, C. H. 2011. "Development of MRI/NIRF 'activatable' multimodal imaging probe based on iron oxide nanoparticles." *J Control Release* 155: 152-158. doi: 10.1016/j.jconrel.2011.07.019.

Chen G. Y., Pang D. W., Hwang S. M., Tuan H. Y., Hu Y. C. 2012. "A graphene-based platform for induced pluripotent stem cells culture and differentiation." *Biomaterials.* 33: 418–427. doi: 10.1016/j.biomaterials.2011.09.071.

Chen Q., Li K., Wen S., Liu H., Peng C., Cai H., 2013. "Targeted CT/MR dual mode imaging of tumors using multifunctional dendrimer-entrapped gold nanoparticles." *Biomaterials* 34: 5200-5209. doi: 10.1016/j.biomaterials.2013.03.009.

Chen Y, Li N, Yang Y, Liu Y. 2015. "A dual targeting cyclodextrin/gold nanoparticle conjugate as a scaffold for solubilization and delivery of paclitaxel." *RSC Adv.* 5: 8938–8941. doi: 10.1039/C4RA13135E.

Cheng, H. L. M., Loai, Y., Beaumont, M., and Farhat, W. A. 2010. "The acellular matrix (ACM) for bladder tissue engineering: a quantitative magnetic resonance imaging study." *Magn Reson Med* 64: 341. doi: 10.1002/mrm.22404.

Deffieux, T., Montaldo, G., Tanter, M., and Fink, M. 2009. "Shear wave spectroscopy for in vivo quantification of human soft tissues visco-elasticity." *IEEE Trans Med Imaging* 28: 313. doi: 10.1109/TMI.2008.925077.

El Fray M, Boccaccini A. R. 2005. "Novel hybrid PET/DFA–TiO2 nanocomposites by in situ polycondensation." *Mater Lett.* 59: 2300–2304. doi: 10.1016/j.matlet.2005.03.008.

Farini, A., Villa, C., Manescu, A., Fiori, F., Giuliani, A., Razini, P., Sitzia, C., Del Fraro, G., Belicchi, M., and Meregalli, M. 2012. "Novel insight into stem cell trafficking in dystrophic muscles." *Int J Nanomed* 7: 3059. doi: 10.2147/IJN.S30595.

Faucher L., Tremblay M., Lagueux J., Gossuin Y., Fortin M. A. 2012. "Rapid synthesis of PEGylated ultrasmall gadolinium oxide nanoparticles for cell labeling and tracking with MRI." *ACS Appl Mater Interfaces* 4: 4506-4515. doi: 10.1021/am3006466.

Feng L., Liu Z. 2011. "Graphene in biomedicine: opportunities and challenges." *Nanomedicine.* 6: 317–324. doi: 10.2217/nnm.10.158.

Fleischmann, D., and Boas, F. E. 2011. "Computed tomography— old ideas and new technology." *Eur Radiol* 21: 510-517. doi: 10.1007/s00330-011-2056-z.

Furno F., Morley K. S., Wong B., Sharp, B. L., Arnold, S. P., Howdle, S. M., Bayston, R., Brown, P. D., Winship, P. D., Reid, H. L. 200. "Silver nanoparticles and polymeric medical devices: a new approach to prevention of infection?" *J Antimicrob Chemother.* 54: 1019–1024. doi: 10.1093/jac/dkh478.

Garra, B. S. 2007. "Imaging and estimation of tissue elasticity by ultrasound." *Ultrasound Q* 23: 255. doi: 10.1097/ruq.0b013e31815b7 ed6.

Giuliani, A., Moroncini, F., Mazzoni, S., Belicchi, M. L., Villa, C., Erratico, S., Colombo, E., Calcaterra, F., Brambilla, L., Torrente, Y., Albertini, G., and Bella, S. D. 2014. "Polyglycolic acid-polylactic acid scaffold response to different progenitor cell in vitro cultures: a demonstrative and comparative X-ray synchrotron radiation phase-contrast microtomography study." *Tissue Eng Part C Methods* 20: 308. doi: 10.1089/ten.tec.2013.0213.

Gonçalves E. M., Oliveira F. J., Silva R. F., Neto, M. A., Fernandes, M. H., Amaral, M., Vallet-Regi, M., Vila, M. 2016. "Three-dimensional printed PCL-hydroxyapatite scaffolds filled with CNTs for bone cell growth stimulation." *J Biomed Mater Res B Appl Biomater.*104: 1210–1219. doi: 10.1002/jbm.b.33432.

Gudur, M., Rao, R. R., Hsiao, Y. S., Peterson, A. W., Deng, C. X. and Stegemann, J. P. 2012. "Non-invasive, quantitative, spatiotemporal characterization of mineralization in three dimensional collagen hydrogels using high-resolution spectral ultrasound imaging." *Tissue Eng Part C Methods* 18: 935. doi: 10.1089/ten.tec.2012.0180.

Han Z. J., Rider A. E., Ishaq M, Kumar, S., Kondyurin, A., Bilek, M. M. M., Levchenko, I., Ostrikov, K. 2013. "Carbon nanostructures for hard tissue engineering." *RSC Adv.* 3: 11058–11072. doi: 10.1039/C2RA23306A.

Hao R., Xing R., Xu Z., Hou Y., Gao S., Sun S. 2010. "Synthesis, functionalization, and biomedical applications of multifunctional magnetic nanoparticles." *Adv Mater.* 22: 2729-2742. doi: 10.1002/adma.201000260.

Harris L., Goff J. D., Carmichael A. Y., Riffle J. S., Harburn J. J., Pierre T. G., Saunders M. 2003. "Magnetite nanoparticle dispersions stabilized with triblock copolymers." *Chem Mater.* 15: 1367–1377. doi: 10.1021/cm020994n.

Hasan A., Morshed, M., Memic, A., Hassan, S., Webster, T. J. and Marei, H. S. 2018. Nanoparticles in tissue engineering: applications, challenges and prospects, *International Journal of Nanomedicine,* 13, 5637–5655. doi: 10.2147/IJN.S153758.

Heo D. N., Ko W. K., Bae M. S., Lee, J. B., Lee, D. W., Byun, W., Lee, C. H., Kim, E. C., Jung, B. Y., Kwon, I. K. 2014. "Enhanced bone regeneration with a gold nanoparticle-hydrogel complex." *J Mater Chem B.* 2: 1584–1593. doi: 10.1039/C3TB21246G.

Hu F., Jia Q., Li Y., Gao M. 2011. "Facile synthesis of ultra-small PEGylated iron oxide nanoparticles for dual-contrast T1- and T2-weighted magnetic resonance imaging." *Nanotechnology* 22: 245604. doi: 10.1088/0957-4484/22/24/245604/meta.

Huihui Xu, Shadi F., Othman and Richard L. M. 2008. "A review on Monitoring Tissue Engineering Using Magnetic Resonance Imaging." *Journal of bioscience and bioengineering* 106: 515–527. doi: 10.1263/jbb.106.515.

Ino K., Kawasumi T., Ito A., Honda H. 2008. "Plasmid DNA transfection using magnetite cationic liposomes for construction of multilayered geneengineered cell sheet." *Biotechnol Bioeng.* 100: 168–176. doi: 10.1002/bit.21738.

Ito A. and Kamihira M. 2011. "Tissue engineering using magnetite nanoparticles." *Prog Mol Biol Transl Sci.*, 104: 355–395. doi: 10.1016/B978-0-12-416020-0.00009-7.

Ito A., Takahashi T., Kameyama Y., Kawabe Y., Kamihira M. 2008. "Magnetic concentration of a retroviral vector using magnetite cationic liposomes." *Tissue Eng C Methods.* 2008;15(1):57–64. doi: 10.1089/ten.tec.2008.0275.

Jaconi M. 2011. "Nanomedicine: gold nanowires to mend a heart." *Nat Nanotechnol.* 6: 692–693. doi: 10.1038/nnano.2011.195.

Jawad H., Boccaccini A. R., Ali N. N. and Harding S. E. 2011. "Assessment of cellular toxicity of TiO2 nanoparticles for cardiac tissue engineering applications." *Nanotoxicology* 5: 372–380. doi: 10.3109/17435390.2010.516844.

Jawad H., Lyon A. R., Harding, S. E., Ali, N. N., Boccaccini, A. R. 2008. "Myocardial tissue engineering." *Br Med Bull.* 87: 31–47.

Johansson, L., in Principles of Translational Science in Medicine (Second Edition), 2015. Chapter 3.7.3 - Translational Imaging Research, Pages 189-194, Academic press.

Ju Y. M., Yu B., Koob T. J., Moussy, Y., Moussy, F. 2008. "A novel porous collagen scaffold around an implantable biosensor for improving biocompatibility. I. In vitro/ in vivo stability of the scaffold and in vitro sensitivity of the glucose sensor with scaffold." *J Biomed Mater Res A.* 87: 136–146. doi: 10.1002/jbm.a.31756.

Jun, Y. W., Lee, J. H., and Cheon, J. 2008. "Chemical design of nanoparticle probes for high-performance magnetic resonance imaging." *Angew ChemInt Ed Engl* 47: 5122. doi: 10.1002/anie.200701674.

Khan Z. H., Ansari M. S., Salah N. A., Memic, M., Habib, S., Shahawi. M. S. 2011. "COBALT catalyzed-multiwalled carbon nanotubes film sensor for carbon mono-oxide gas." *Dig J Nanomater Biostruct.* 6: 1947-1956.

Khang D., Kim S. Y., Liu-Snyder P, Palmore G. T., Durbin S. M., Webster T. J. 2007. "Enhanced fibronectin adsorption on carbon nanotube/poly (carbonate) urethane: independent role of surface nano-roughness and associated surface energy." *Biomaterials.* 28: 4756–4768. doi: 10.1016/j.biomaterials.2007.07.018.

Kharaziha M., Memic A., Akbari M., Brafman D. A., Nikkhah M. 2016. "Nano-enabled approaches for stem cell-based cardiac tissue engineering." *Adv Healthc Mater.* 5: 1533–1553. doi: 10.1002/adhm. 201600088.

Kim H., Che L., Ha Y., Ryu W. 2014. "Mechanically-reinforced electrospun composite silk fibroin nanofibers containing hydroxyapatite nanoparticles." *Mater Sci Eng C.* 40: 324–335. doi: 10.1016/j.msec.2014.04.012.

Kim J., Kim Y. R., Kim Y. J., Lim, K. T., Seonwoo, H., Park, S., Cho, S. P., Hong, B. H., Choung, P. H., Chung, T. D., Choung, Y. H., and Chung, J. H. 2013. "Graphene-incorporated chitosan substrata for adhesion and differentiation of human mesenchymal stem cells." *J Mater Chem B.* 1: 933–938. doi: 10.1039/C2TB00274D.

Ko W. K., Heo D. N., Moon H. J., 2015. "The effect of gold nanoparticle size on osteogenic differentiation of adipose-derived stem cells." *J Colloid Interface Sci.* 438: 68–76. doi: 10.1016/j.jcis.2014.08.058.

Koo O. M., Rubinstein I, Onyuksel H. 2005. "Role of nanotechnology in targeted drug delivery and imaging: a concise review." *Nanomedicine.* 1: 193–212. doi: 10.1016/j.nano.2005.06.004.

Kreitz, S., Dohmen, G., Hasken, S., Schmitz-Rode, T., Mela, P., and Jockenhoevel, S. 2011. "Nondestructive method to evaluate the collagen content of fibrin-based tissue engineered structures via ultrasound." *Tissue Eng Part C Methods* 17: 1021. doi: 10.1089/ ten.tec.2010.0669.

Krötz F., Sohn H. Y., Gloe T., Plank C., Pohl U. 2003. "Magnetofection potentiates gene delivery to cultured endothelial cells." *J Vasc Res.* 40: 425–434. doi: 10.1159/000073901.

Kubota Y., Shuin T., Kawasaki C., Hosaka, M., Kitamura, H., Cai, R., Sakai, H., Hashimoto, K., Fujishima, A. 1994. "Photokilling of T-24 human bladder cancer cells with titanium dioxide." *Br J Cancer.* 70: 1107–1111. URL: https://www.ncbi.nlm.nih.gov/pmc/articles/PMC2033697/.

Langer R., Vacanti J. P. 1993. "Tissue Engineering." *Science* 260, 920-926. doi: 10.1126/science.8493529.

Lansman J. B. 1990. "Blockade of current through single calcium channels by trivalent lanthanide cations. Effect of ionic radius on the rates of ion entry and exit." *J Gen Physiol* 95: 679-696. doi: 10.1085/jgp.95.4.679.

Laurent S., Forge D., Port M., Roch A., Robic C., Vander Elst L., Muller, R. N. 2008. "Magnetic iron oxide nanoparticles: Synthesis, stabilization, vectorization, physicochemical characterizations, and biological applications." *Chem Rev* 108: 2064. doi: 10.1021/cr06 8445e.

Lee C. H., Kim E. Y., Jeon K., Tae, J. C., Lee, K. S., Kim, Y. O., Jeong, M. Y., Yun, C. W., Jeong, D. K., Cho, S. K., Kim, J. H., Lee, H. Y., Riu, K. Z., Cho, S. G., Park, S. P. 2008. "Simple, efficient, and reproducible gene transfection of mouse embryonic stem cells by magnetofection." *Stem Cells Dev.* 17: 133–142. doi: 10.1089/scd.200 7.0064.

Li N., Fan X., Tang K., Zheng X., Liu J., Wang B. 2016. "Nanocomposite scaffold with enhanced stability by hydrogen bonds between collagen, polyvinyl pyrrolidone and titanium dioxide." *Colloids Surf B Biointerfaces.* 140: 287–296. doi: 10.1016/j.colsurfb.2015.12.005.

Lim D., Lee E., Kim H., Park S., Baek S., Yoon J. 2015. "Multi stimuli-responsive hydrogel microfibers containing magnetite nanoparticles prepared using microcapillary devices." *Soft Matter.* 11: 1606–1613. doi: 10.1039/C4SM02564D.

Lim J. S., Kook M. S., Jung S., et al. 2014. "Plasma treated high-density polyethylene (HDPE) medpor implant immobilized with rhBMP-2 for improving the bone regeneration." *J Nanomater.* 2014:7. doi: 10.5555/ 2677685.2677691.

Liu A., Hong Z., Zhuang X., Chen, X., Cui, Y., Liu, Y., Jing, X. 2008. "Surface modification of bioactive glass nanoparticles and the mechanical and biological properties of poly (L-lactide) composites." *Acta Biomater.* 4: 1005–1015. doi: 10.1016/j.actbio.2008.02.013.

Liu D., Zhang J. C., Yi C. Q., Yang M. S. 2010. "The effects of gold nanoparticles on the proliferation, differentiation, and mineralization function of MC3T3-E1 cells in vitro." *Chin Sci Bull.* 55: 1013–1019. doi: 10.1007/s11434-010-0046-1

Liu H., Slamovich E. B., Webster T. J. 2006. "Less harmful acidic degradation of poly(lactic-co-glycolic acid) bone tissue engineering scaffolds through titania nanoparticle addition." *Int J Nanomed.* 1: 541–545. url: https://www.ncbi.nlm.nih.gov/pmc/articles/PMC2676635/.

Luderer F., Begerow I., Schmidt W., Martin, H., Grabow, N., Bunger, C. M., Schareck, W., Schmitz, K. P., Stemberg, K. 2013. "Enhanced visualization of biodegradable polymeric vascular scaffolds by incorporation of gold, silver and magnetite nanoparticles." *J Biomater Appl.* 28: 219–231. doi: 10.1177/0885328212443393.

Magiera A., Markowski J., Menaszek E., Pilch, J., Blazewicz, S. 2017. "PLA-based hybrid and composite electrospun fibrous scaffolds as potential materials for tissue engineering." *J Nanomater.* 2017: 11. doi: 10.1155/2017/9246802.

Mankoff D. A. 2007. "A definition of molecular imaging." *J Nucl Med* 48: 18N-21N. URL: http://jnm.snmjournals.org/content/48/6/18N.long.

Mironov V., Kasyanov V., Markwald R. R. 2008. "Nanotechnology in vascular tissue engineering: from nanoscaffolding towards rapid vessel biofabrication." *Trends Biotechnol.* 26: 338–344. doi: 10.1016/j.tibtech.2008.03.001.

Nam, S. Y., Ricles, L. M., B. S., Suggs, S. J., and Emelianov, S. Y. 2014. "Imaging Strategies for Tissue Engineering Applications." *Tissue engineering: Part B*, 21; 115. doi: 10.1089/ten.teb.2014.0180.

Nanotechnology in Tissue Engineering. WWW.azonano.com, 2017.

Navaei A., Saini H., Christenson W., Sullivan R. T., Ros R., Nikkhah M. 2016. "Gold nanorod-incorporated gelatin-based conductive hydrogels for engineering cardiac tissue constructs." *Acta Biomater.* 41: 133–146. doi: 10.1016/j.actbio.2016.05.027.

Neuberger T., Schöpf B., Hofmann H., Hofmann, M., Rechenberg, B. 2005. "Superparamagnetic nanoparticles for biomedical applications: possibilities and limitations of a new drug delivery system." *J Magn Magn Mater.* 293: 483–496. doi: 10.1016/j.jmmm.2005.01.064.

Ntziachristos, V. 2010. "Going deeper than microscopy: the optical imaging frontier in biology." *Nat Methods* 7: 603. doi: 10.1038/nmeth.1483.

Pan L, Pei X, He R, Wan Q, Wang J. 2012. "Multiwall carbon nanotubes/polycaprolactone composites for bone tissue engineering application." *Colloids Surf B Biointerfaces.* 2012;93:226–234. doi: 10.1016/j.colsurfb.2012.01.011.

Papantoniou, I., Sonnaert, M., Geris, L., Luyten, F. P., Schrooten, J., and Kerckhofs, G. 2014. "Three-dimensional characterization of tissue-engineered constructs by contrast enhanced Nano focus computed tomography." *Tissue Eng Part C Methods* 20: 177. doi: 10.1089/ten.TEC.2013.0041.

Park J. A., Kim H. K., Kim J. H., Jeong S. W., Jung J. C., Lee G. H., Lee J., Chang Y., Kim T. J. 2010. "Gold nanoparticles functionalized by gadolinium DTPA conjugate of cysteine as a multimodal bio-imaging agent." *Bioorg Med Chem Lett.* 20: 2287-2291. doi: 10.1016/j.bmcl.2010.02.002.

Pittenger M. F., Mackay A. M., Beck S. C., Jaiswall, R. K., Douglas, R., Moscal, J. D., Moormanl, M. A., Simonettil, D. W., Craig, S., Marshak, D. R. 1999. "Multilineage potential of adult human mesenchymal stem cells." *Science* 284: 143–147. doi: 10.1126/science.284.5411.143.

Radomska A, Leszczyszyn J, Radomski M. W. 2016. "The nanopharmacology and nanotoxicology of nanomaterials: new opportunities and challenges." *Adv Clin Exp Med.* 25: 151–162. doi: 10.17219/acem/60879.

Ramaswamy, S., Wang, D. A., Fishbein, K. W., Elisseeff, J. H., and Spencer, R. G. 2006. "An analysis of the integration between articular cartilage and non-degradable hydrogel using magnetic resonance imaging." *J Biomed Mater Res Part B Appl Biomater* 77: 144. doi: 10.1002/jbm.b.30404.

Ravichandran R, Sridhar R, Venugopal JR, Sundarrajan S, Mukherjee S, Ramakrishna S. 2014. "Gold nanoparticle loaded hybrid nanofibers for cardiogenic differentiation of stem cells for infarcted myocardium regeneration." *Macromol Biosci.* 14: 515–525. doi: 10.1002/mabi.201300407.

Ravichandran R., Sridhar R., Venugopal J. R., Sundarrajan S., Mukherjee S., Ramakrishna S. 2014. "Gold nanoparticle loaded hybrid nanofibers for cardiogenic differentiation of stem cells for infarcted myocardium regeneration." *Macromol Biosci.* 14: 515–525. doi: 10.1002/mabi.201300407

Rodríguez-Lozano F. J., García-Bernal D., Aznar-Cervantes S., Oñate-Sánchez R. E., Moraleda J. M. 2015. "Potential of graphene for tissue engineering applications." *Transl Res.* 166: 399–400. doi: 10.1016/j.trsl.2015.04.003.

Scherer F., Anton M., Schillinger U., Henke, J., Bergemann, C., Krüger, A., Gänsbacher B., Plank, C. 2002. "Magnetofection: enhancing and targeting gene delivery by magnetic force in vitro and in vivo." *Gene Ther.* 9:102-109. doi: 10.1038/sj.gt.3301624.

Shellock F. G., Kanal E. 1999. "Safety of magnetic resonance imaging contrast agents." *J Magn Reson Imaging* 10: 477-484. doi: 10.1002/(SICI)1522-2586(199909)10:3<477::AID-JMRI33>3.0.CO;2-E.

Shevach M., Fleischer S., Shapira A., Dvir T. 2014. "Gold nanoparticle-decellularized matrix hybrids for cardiac tissue engineering." *Nano Lett.* 14: 5792–5796. doi: 10.1021/nl502673m.

Shevach M., Maoz B. M., Feiner R., Shapira, A., Dvir, T. 2013. "Nanoengineering gold particle composite fibers for cardiac tissue engineering." *J Mater Chem B.* 1: 5210–5217. doi: 10.1039/C3TB20584C.

Shi J., Votruba A. R., Farokhzad O. C., Langer R. 2010. "Nanotechnology in drug delivery and tissue engineering: from discovery to applications." *Nano Lett.* 10: 3223–3230. doi: 10.1021/nl102184c.

Shin S. R., Shin C., Memic A., Shadmehr, S., Miscuglio, M., Jung, H. Y., Jung, S. M., Bae, H., Khademhosseini, A., Tang, X., Dokmeci, M. R. 2015. "Aligned carbon nanotube–based flexible gel substrates for engineering biohybrid tissue actuators." *Adv Funct Mater.* 25: 4486–4495. doi: 10.1002/adfm.201501379.

Smirnov P., Lavergne E., Gazeau F., Lewin M., Boissonnas A., Doan B. T., Gillet, B., Combadière, C., Combadière, B., Clément, O. 2006. "In vivo cellular imaging of lymphocyte trafficking by MRI: A tumor model approach to cell-based anticancer therapy." *Magn Reson Med.* 56: 498-508. doi: 10.1002/mrm.20996.

Stout D. A., Basu B., Webster T. J. 2011. "Poly (lactic-co-glycolic acid): carbon nanofiber composites for myocardial tissue engineering applications." *Acta Biomater.* 7: 3101–3112. doi: 10.1016/j.actbio. 2011.04.028.

Subbiah R., Veerapandian M., Yun K. S. 2010. "Nanoparticles: functionalization and multifunctional applications in biomedical sciences." *Curr Med Chem.* 17: 4559–4577. doi: 10.2174/09298671 0794183024.

Suh K. S., Lee Y. S., Seo S. H., Kim Y. S., Choi E. M. 2013. "Gold nanoparticles attenuates antimycin A-induced mitochondrial dysfunction in MC3T3-E1 osteoblastic cells." *Biol Trace Elem Res.* 153: 428–436. doi: 10.1007/s12011-013-9679-7.

Tanaka, Y., Saijo, Y., Fujihara, Y., Yamaoka, H., Nishizawa, S., Nagata, S., Ogasawara, T., Asawa, Y., Takato, T., and Hoshi, K. 2012. "Evaluation of the implant type tissue engineered cartilage by scanning acoustic microscopy." *J Biosci Bioeng* 113: 252. doi: 10.1016/j.jbiosc. 2011.10.011.

Terreno, E., Delli Castelli, D., Viale, A., and Aime, S. 2010. "Challenges for molecular magnetic resonance imaging." *Chem Rev* 110: 3019. doi: 10.1021/cr100025t.

Thimm, B. W., Hofmann, S., Schneider, P., Carretta, R., and Mu ̈ller, R. 2011. "Imaging of cellular spread on a three-dimensional scaffold by means of a novel cell-labelling technique for high-resolution computed tomography." *Tissue Eng Part C Methods* 18: 167. doi: 10.1089/ten. tec.2011.0262.

Tran P. A., Zhang L., Webster T J. 2009. "Carbon nanofibers and carbon nanotubes in regenerative medicine." *Adv. Drug Del. Rev.* 61: 1097 – 1114. doi: 10.1016/j.addr.2009.07.010.

Wang Q and Chen D. 2016. "Synthesis and characterization of a chitosan based nanocomposite injectable hydrogel." *Carbohydr Polym.* 136: 1228–1237. doi: 10.1016/j.carbpol.2015.10.040.

Wang S., Castro R., An X., Song, C., Luo, Y., Shen, M., Tomas, H., Zhu, M., and Shi, X. 2012. "Electrospun laponite-doped poly (lactic-co-glycolic acid) nanofibers for osteogenic differentiation of human mesenchymal stem cells." *J Mater Chem.* 22: 23357–23367. doi: 10.1039/C2JM34249A.

Wang, Y., Bella, E., Lee, C. S., Migliaresi, C., Pelcastre, L., Schwartz, Z., Boyan, B. D. and Motta, A. 2010. "The synergistic effects of 3-D porous silk fibroin matrix scaffold properties and hydrodynamic environment in cartilage tissue regeneration." *Biomaterials* 31: 4672. doi: 10.1016/j.biomaterials.2010.02.006.

Wanjale S. D., Jog J. P. 2006. "Crystallization and phase transformation kinetics of poly (1-butene)/MWCNT nanocomposites." *Polymer.* 47: 6414–6421. doi: 10.1016/j.polymer.2006.07.011.

Wells P. N. T., and Liang, H. D. 2011. "Medical ultrasound: imaging of soft tissue strain and elasticity." *J R Soc Interface* 8: 1521. doi: 10.1098/rsif.2011.0054.

Wen S., Li K., Cai H., Chen Q., Shen M., Huang Y., Peng C., Hou W., Zhu M., Zhang G., Shi X. 2013. "Multifunctional dendrimer-entrapped gold nanoparticles for dual mode CT/MR imaging applications." *Biomaterials* 34: 1570-1580. doi: 10.1016/j.biomaterials.2012.11.010.

Wilson D. S., Dalmasso G., Wang L., Sitaraman S. V., Merlin D., Murthy N. 2010. "Orally delivered thioketal nanoparticles loaded with TNF-alpha-siRNA target inflammation and inhibit gene expression in the intestines." *Nat Mater.* 9: 923–928. doi: 10.1038/NMAT2859.

Winterroth, F., Hollman, K. W., Kuo, S., Izumi, K., Feinberg, S. E., Hollister, S. J., and Fowlkes, J. B. 2011. "Comparison of scanning acoustic microscopy and histology images in characterizing surface irregularities among engineered human oral mucosal tissues." *Ultrasound Med Biol* 37: 1734. doi: 10.1016/j.ultrasmedbio.2011.06.010.

Winterroth, F., Hollman, K.W., Kuo, S., Ganguly, A., Feinberg, S. E., Fowlkes, J. B., and Hollister, S. J. 2012. "Characterizing morphology and nonlinear elastic properties of normal and thermally stressed engineered oral mucosal tissues using scanning acoustic microscopy." *Tissue Eng Part C Methods* 19: 345. doi: 10.1089/ten.tec.2012.0467.

Xie H., Zhu Y., Jiang W., Zhou Q., Yang H., Gu N., Zhang Y. Xu H., Xu H., Yang X. 2011. "Lactoferrin-conjugated superparamagnetic iron oxide nanoparticles as a specific MRI contrast agent for detection of brain glioma in vivo." *Biomaterials* 32: 495-502. doi: 10.1016/ j.biomaterials.2010.09.024.

Xu W., Park J. Y., Kattel K., Ahmad M. W., Bony B. A., Heo W. C., Jin S., Park J. W., Chang Y., Kim T. J., Park J. A., Do J. Y., Chae K. S., Lee G. H. 2012. "Fluorescein-polyethyleneimine coated gadolinium oxide nanoparticles as T 1 magnetic resonance imaging (MRI)–cell labeling (CL) dual agents." *RSC Adv.* 2: 10907-10915. doi: 10.1039/ C2RA21052E.

Yadollahpour A. 2015. "Magnetic nanoparticles in medicine: A review of synthesis methods and important characteristics." *Oriental J Chem* 31: 271-277. doi: 10.13005/ojc/31.Special-Issue1.33.

Yadollahpour A., Hosseini S. A., Jalilifar M., Rashidi S., Rai B. M. 2016. "Magnetic nanoparticle-based drug and gene delivery: A review of recent advances and clinical applications." *Int J Pharm Technol.* 8: 11451-11466.

Yadollahpour A., Jalilifar M, Rashidi S. 2016. "A review of the feasibility and clinical applications of magnetic nanoparticles as contrast agents in magnetic resonance imaging." *Int J Pharm Technol.* 8: 14737-14748. URL: http://www.ijptonline.com/wp-content/uploads/2016/10/ 14737-14748.pdf.

Yadollahpour A., Rashidi S. 2015. "Magnetic nanoparticles: A review of chemical and physical characteristics important in medical applications." *Oriental J Chem.* 31: 25-30.

Yadollahpour A., Venkateshwarlu G. 2016. "Applications of gadolinium nanoparticles in magnetic resonance imaging: A review on recent advances in clinical imaging." *Int J Pharm Technol.* 8: 11379-11393.

Yadollahpour, A., Mansoury, H., Rashidi, S. 2017. "Applications of Nanoparticles in Magnetic Resonance Imaging: A Comprehensive Review." *Asian Journal of Pharmaceutics* 11: S7. URL: http://www.asiapharmaceutics.info/index.php/ajp/article/view/1083.

Yang H., Zhuang Y., Sun Y., Dai A., Shi X., Wu D., Li F., Hu H., Yang S. 2011. "Targeted dual-contrast T1- and T2-weighted magnetic resonance imaging of tumors using multifunctional gadolinium-labeled superparamagnetic iron oxide nanoparticles." *Biomaterials* 32: 4584-93. doi: 10.1016/j.biomaterials.2011.03.018.

Yu, J., Takanari, K., Hong, Y., Lee, K.-W., Amoroso, N.J., Wang, Y., Wagner, W.R., and Kim, K. 2013. "Non-invasive characterization of polyurethane-based tissue constructs in a rat abdominal repair model using high frequency ultrasound elasticity imaging." *Biomaterials* 34: 2701. doi: 10.1016/j.biomaterials.2013.01.036.

Zhang B., Jin H., Li Y., Chen B., Liu S., Shi D. 2012. "Bioinspired synthesis of gadolinium-based hybrid nanoparticles as MRI blood pool contrast agents with high relaxivity." *J Mater Chem* 22: 14494-14501. doi: 10.1039/C2JM30629H.

Zhang H. W., Wang L. Q., Xiang Q. F., Zhong Q., Chen L. M., Xu C. X., Xiang X. H., Xu B., Meng F., Wan Y. Q., Deng D. Y. B. 2014. "Specific lipase-responsive polymer-coated gadolinium nanoparticles for MR imaging of early acute pancreatitis." *Biomaterials* 35: 356-367. doi: 10.1016/j.biomaterials.2013.09.046.

In: Nanoparticles ISBN: 978-1-53616-596-8
Editors: A. K. Samantara, S. Ratha

Chapter 5

NANOMEDICINE: AN ALTERNATIVE TO CONVENTIONAL DIAGNOSTIC AND THERAPEUTIC OPTIONS IN ORAL CANCER

***Lora Mishra*[1,*] *and Satyaranjan Misra*[2]**
[1]Department of Conservative Dentistry and Endontics,
Institute of Dental Sciences, Siksha 'O' Anusandhan University,
Bhubaneswar, Odisha, India
[2]Department of Oral Medicine and Radiology,
Institute of Dental Sciences, Siksha 'O' Anusandhan University,
Bhubaneswar, Odisha, India

ABSTRACT

Oral carcinoma is an aggressive cancer with significant social stigma and a high recurrence rate. Prompt diagnosis is of paramount importance for preventing oral cancer and its management. Biopsy, though an invasive and painful procedure, remains the gold standard for diagnosis. Few non-invasive methods like vital staining, scrape cytology and molecular diagnostic methods have poor sensitivity and specificity.

* Corresponding Author's Email: loramishra@soa.ac.in.

Similarly the use of chemotherapeutic agents in oral cancer has limited effect due to its toxic side effects and poor efficacy. Hence, there is a dire requirement for finding non-invasive, greatly sensitive, and highly specific detection techniques. Nanotechnology based detection systems increase the sensitivity of the biomarkers to a nano-scale. Nanotechnology provides a substitute to conventional anti-cancer therapy that leads to increased efficiency and decrease in toxicity. The use of nano-based diagnostic and therapeutic systems may be a promising means to show real-time, easy to use, and affordable diagnostic imaging and treatment which specifically acts on the malignant cells thereby being safe and efficacious.

Keywords: local drug delivery, nanotechnology, novel diagnostic techniques, oral cancer

1. INTRODUCTION

Oral cancer (OSCC; oral squamous cell carcinoma) is the most prevalent malignancies in the head and neck region, associated with morbidity and mortality. In spite of measures at improving prompt diagnosis and treatment, there is a poor 5-year survival rate associated with the disease which significantly increases the oral cancer burden worldwide (Siegel et al. 2016, 7). Newer approaches to minimise diagnostic pitfalls and enhance therapeutic protocols pave the path of research in oral cancer (Calixto et al. 2014, 3719). Nano-medicine has emerged as a novel platform for diagnostic and therapeutic advances in oral cancer (Torre et al. 2012, 87). Many clinical trials are underway for providing efficient MRI contrast agents used in the staging of the disease and targeted drug therapies using different delivery systems to enhance the efficacy and tolerability of drugs (Tanaka and Ishigamori 2011, 603740). When nano-platforms are used for chemotherapeutic agents, there can be significant rise in the anti-neoplastic activity of the drug even when the cells are chemo-resistant when the drug is used singly with a reduced toxicity to the patients (Warnakulasuriya 2009, 309). It has also been observed that the effect of photodynamic and gene therapies increases on using targeted magnetic nanoparticles with inhibition of gene expression. The future research in the diagnosis and treatment of oral cancer is aimed at developing more nanoparticle-based drug delivery systems and to assess the potency of nanoparticle-based therapies both *in vitro* and *in vivo* (Ng et al. 2017, 297; Jemal et al. 2011, 69; Arakeri et al. 2017, 413).

2. Nanotechnology Based Diagnostic Modalities for Oral Cancer

Novel diagnostic modalities are the need of the hour to create good clinical outcomes and better prognosis, by accurate predication of the malignant potential of oral potentially malignant disorders (OPMDs), diagnosis of oral carcinoma using molecular targeting, nano scale ultra-sensitive diagnostic strategies, real time recommendations regarding surgical resection margins and post treatment follow-up of oral cancer for easy monitoring (Benergossi et al. 2015, 345; Liu et al. 2016, 165). Nanotechnology has been successfully used in the detection of oral cancer using various imaging modalities (Figure 1).

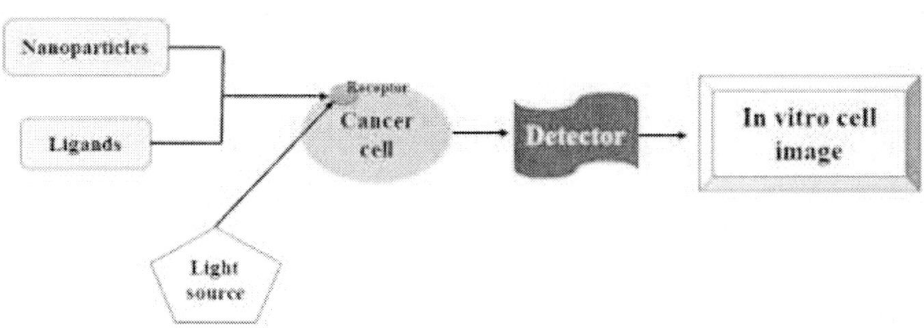

Figure 1. Nanoparticle based bio-imaging in oral cancer.

2.1. Magnetic Resonance Imaging

Magnetic resonance imaging (MRI) is the detection method of choice for the discovery of the primary tumour and the soft tissue invasion as well as lymph-node metastasis in oral carcinomas (Sarrion Perez et al. 2015, 1880). It is also used for delineating the tumour margins intra-operatively and in the post-operative follow-up to rule out recurrence. Gadolinium-based contrast agents are commonly used for MRI. But these contrast agents are not tumour specific and disseminate through the blood circulation to the entire body after intra-venous injections (Hinni et al. 2013, 1190). Moreover, these contrast agents have a short half-life period of about one to two hours in the blood circulation. The contrast agents are made up of superparamagnetic nanoparticles which have layers of coatings on them. As the technology of nanoparticles improved, specific MRI contrast agents for oral cancer screening are available (Cheng 2013, 23). These newer nano-contrast agents are capable of recognizing unique markers on the cell surface have a better half-life in the blood circulation and hence enhanced contrast properties in MRI (Brigger et al. 2002, 631).

Magnetic poly (lactide-co-glycolide) (PLGA) nanoparticles and folate preconjugated chitosan were used by Asifkhan et al. to fabricate a new MRI contrast agent especially for oral carcinoma (Shanavas et al. 2017, 112). It was seen that the T2 relaxation time became shorter enhancing the contrast due to increase in relaxivity of the nanoparticles. The oral cancer cells which were folate receptor positive exhibited enhanced uptake of nanoparticles thus causing significant increase in cytotoxicity. Hence this nanoparticle agent was not only diagnostic with high contrast imaging of cancer but it also simultaneously provided therapeutic benefits in oral cancer (Chandran et al. 2011, 4150). Yet another unique magnetic nanoparticle-based contrast agent was developed on Gadolinium doped amorphous Titanium dioxide which is useful for T1 weighted MR images. The capability to induce hemolysis, platelet aggregation as well as plasma coagulation was investigated and no adverse reactions were reported (Chandran et al. 2011, 4150). Therefore folic acid conjugated nanoparticles were distinctly clustered on the oral cancer KB cells which were folate receptor positive. Such nanoparticle contrast agent exhibited increased longitudinal relaxivity, good biocompatibility and imaging for MRI.

2.2. Optical Coherence Tomography

Optical coherence tomography (OCT) is a unique imaging technique which directly simulates ultrasonography. It is capable of producing cross-sectional anatomical images of the tissues below the oral mucosa like the epithelium and the basement membrane with the use of infra-red light which can penetrate about 2 mm below the oral mucosa (Green et al. 2016, 180). Hence it can be used to detect dysplastic changes in oral potentially malignant disorders and prompt diagnosis of oral cancer. OCT has a resolution of about 10 μm which is greater than that of other imaging modalities like CT, MRI, and ultrasound. In spite of being able to provide real-time data regarding the cellular and stromal morphology and being non-invasive, it is handicapped with poor contrast between the normal and malignant neoplastic tissues (Kah et al. 2007, 785).

Recently due to excellent biocompatibility, ease of synthesis and ability to provide at infra-red wavelengths local surface plasmon resonance which are not absorbed by the tissues, gold nanoparticles are used as effective OCT contrast agents (Kim et al. 2009, 034008). The Epidermal growth factor receptor (EGFR) monoclonal antibodies conjugated gold nanoparticles having a diameter of 71 nm were used to increase the contrast of oral dysplastic images in OCT in animal models. To enhance the delivery of the particles into the mucosal surface ultrasound and microneedles were used and this resulted in about 150% increase in the contrast level (Kim et al. 2009, 034008; Oldenburg et al. 2006, 6724).

2.3. Photoacoustic Imaging

Another emerging imaging modality is photoacoustic imaging, which uses short LASER pulses, and generates transient ultrasound impulses from tissues, causing temporary thermos-elastic expansions after absorbing the LASER energy (Bayer et al. 2017, 757; Zhang et al. 2016, 1920). These thermo-elastic changes are then converted into photoacoustic images depending on the time of the impulse received by an ultrasound transducer (Xu et al. 2018, 56). Such images have good spatial resolution for morphologic evaluation and are very useful in detecting lymph node metastasis especially post-surgery (Jiang et al. 2017, 1700710). Also the photo acoustic imaging can give imaging depth to about 6 cm and using gold nanoparticles as a contrast agent is promising due to the ability of conjugation of biomolecules subsequently producing stronger photo acoustic imaging signals (Liang et al. 2015, 970).

Luke et al. investigated metastatic murine models of OSCC using ultrasound-guided spectroscopic photoacoustic imaging modality to detect lymph node micro-metastases (Luke et al. 2016, 5397). When anti-EGFR antibody was conjugated with molecularly activated plasmonic nanosensors (MAPS), it has been seen that the MAPS shifted their absorption spectra to the near-infrared region. Besides in micro-metastases of about 50 nm good ultrasound-guided spectroscopic photoacoustic signals appeared within half an hour of a MAPS injection (Luke et al. 2016, 5397). This novel method could be used as a substitute to the biopsy of the sentinel lymph nodes in the surgical interventions for oral carcinoma.

2.4. Surface Plasmon Resonance Scattering

The sum of the oscillations of conducting electrons in noble metals creates surface plasmon waves (Hou et al. 2017, 24126). Out of others the gold nanoparticles are broadly studied for this purpose. Gold nanoparticles employed recently for surface plasmon resonance scattering because gold nanoparticles resonantly scattered near-infrared and visible light because of their surface plasmon oscillation (Sokolov et al. 2013, 1999). Besides preparing gold nanoparticles is simpler, they have low cytotoxicity and are easily bi-conjugated, thus enabling them viable for labelling and targeting of biomolecules (Hou et al. 2017, 24126). Since conjugated nanoparticles cluster together, they induce a vastly increased surface plasmon resonance scattering when compared to the unconjugated nanoparticles. Surface plasmon resonance absorption spectra and scattering images after cell incubation were described by El-sayeed et al. (El-Sayed et al. 2005, 829). They concluded that the EGFR conjugated nanoparticles specifically attach onto the surface of the malignant cells at a greater concentration but the binding to the non-malignant cells was haphazard and meagre as observed in light scattering images (El-Sayed et al. 2005, 829). It was also seen that the surface plasmon resonance ability of gold nanoparticles increased Raman scattering in the salivary samples of oral carcinoma patients. The gold nanoparticles aggregated near the target malignant cells; because they were conjugated with anti-EGFR and enhanced the surface plasmon resonance producing high optic signals (Kah et al. 2007, 785).

2.5. Surface-Enhanced Raman Spectroscopy

Raman spectroscopy is a spectroscopic vibrational technique which is based on inelastic interactions between matter and light (Yan et al. 2015, 650). The normal, potentially malignant and malignant oral lesions are differentiated by inelastic scattering of light by LASERS, in the range of visible, near-ultraviolet or near-infrared spectra (Harmsen et al. 2017, 1400). These signals reflect the changes in the chemical characteristics and molecular architecture of the tissues, with homogenous signals from normal tissues and heterogeneous in malignant cells (Guze et al. 2015, 511). But the drawback of the Raman spectroscopy was low penetration depth and low signal intensity resulting in a near field effect (Liu et al. 2017, 38222). However, addition of nanoparticles exogenously as contrast agents for acquiring Raman signal with high resolution and speed is gaining importance. So direct adsorption on the surface of the nanoparticles leads to the emission of an amplified intensity of Raman scattering, called surface-enhanced Raman scattering (SERS) (Guze et al. 2015, 511). When small, round, near-infrared region sensitive, SERS active gold nano-particles were introduced with very small intra-nanogap structures in solitary oral carcinoma cell imaging, the gold nano-particles specifically targeted cell organelles which were particularly scattered through-out the cytoplasm, mitochondria, and nuclei, resulting in great speed Raman imaging in a short time with high resolution images (Liu et al. 2017, 38222).

Gold nanoparticles can exist in different morphologies as spheres, rods, cubes, branches, pyramids, etc. Due to higher index sensitivity of gold nanorods (GNRs) small changes in the near environment results in high longitudinal surface plasmon resonance peak wavelength variation and is of much use in molecular imaging (Kang et al. 2015, 1766). The longitudinal plasmon wavelengths and index sensitivity of nanorods is greatly enhanced with the size of the aspect ratios, hence the utilization of nanorods with high aspect ratios are recommended for providing near-infrared region plasmon wavelengths and greater index sensitivity (El-Sayeed et al. 2015, 829).

Wang et al. have conjugated a dye (RB; rose Bengal) to the gold nanoparticle surface and observed an optical absorption in the near infrared region (Wang et al. 2013, 4274). As the molecules of the RB dye bind to the nucleic acid or protein in malignant cell lysate, aggregation of RB-GNR probes could provide a sensitive and quantifying method for oral cancer cell lysate analysis (Chen et al. 2008, 5233). In a study using SERS technology by Liu et al. oral epithelial cells obtained after exfoliative cytology, were spread on a plasmonic paper adsorbed with GNRs and the spectra were obtained for the cells (Wang et al. 2013, 4274). It was seen that there was 100% specificity and sensitivity in distinguishing between the normal and malignant tissues based on the exfoliation of cells, overcoming the drawbacks of conventional exfoliative cytology (Wang et al. 2013, 4274).

2.6. Diffusion Reflection Imaging

Diffusion reflection imaging is an imaging modality in which, a minute portion of visible light penetrating the living tissue is either transmitted or absorbed and the remaining encounters numerous elastic scattering getting reflected widely (Liu et al. 2014, 128). This reflected light is significantly affected by cyto-architectural and histo-morphologic changes like epithelial dysplasia, size of the nucleus, content of collagen, structure of the cellular matrix, width of epithelial cells and the vascularity of the lamina propria (Chen et al. 2015, 87). Diffuse reflectance images can aid in delineating surgical margins, thereby proving its use in differentiating between normal oral mucosa, oral potentially malignant disorder and oral carcinoma.

Identification of tumour margins in OSCC is a challenge and correct delineation of the margins is critical for adequate surgical resection of residual malignant cells to reduce the high recurrent rate associated with OSCC (Jayanthi 2011, 000071). Frozen sections are generally used with routine microscopy intra-operatively but the shrinkage of the frozen tissues limits its accuracy. Hence in a study by Ankri et al. (2016, 2349) monoclonal antibodies attached with GNRs against EGFR were employed and human OSCC specimen margins were evaluated by diffusion reflection imaging (DFI) (Tasche et al. 2017, 1166). The GNRs-EGFR were scattered at a length of 1 mm between the malignant and the normal regions as observed in scanning electron microscopy images. DFI conducted in the 1mm resolution, showed the tumour margins in a 4–5 mm range, which is in agreement with the accepted cut off of 5 mm for narrow margins. The sensitivity was 87% and the specificity was 97%, while the reflectance spectrum was moderate in carcinoma in situ cases, but deficient in healthy epithelium at 780 nm (Ankri et al. 2016, 2349). It was also seen that reflectance intensity increased with an increase in the dysplastic changes and hence this technique could be useful both for screening of oral malignancy as well as in the detection of residual malignant disease intra-operatively.

2.7. Quantum Dots Imaging

Table 1. Advantages and disadvantages of different imaging modalities using nanotechnology (Xiao-Jie et al. 2018, 52)

Imaging Modality	Advantages	Disadvantages
Magnetic Resonance Imaging	Nano-contrast agents have longer retention in the blood stream and enhance image contrast.	High cost
Optical Coherence Tomography	Nano-contrast agents have 150% better contrast and biocompatible.	Limited penetration depth with technique sensitive operation.
Photoacoustic Imaging	Nano-sensors give larger photoacoustic signals.	Difficult real time imaging.
Surface-enhanced Raman Scattering	Nanorods having high aspect ratios show near infra-red region plasmon wavelength with high index sensitivity.	Limited availability of nanomaterials with sers effect and difficult to prepare probes.
Surface Plasmon Resonance Scattering	Gold nanoparticles may resonantly scatter near-infrared and visible light by virtue of surface plasmon oscillation.	Difficulty in achieving stability of the nanoparticles.
Quantom Dot's Imaging	High fluorescence intensity, good specificity and stability.	Cytotoxicity and biodegradability issues to be addressed.
Diffusion Reflection Imaging	Gold-nanorods useful for oral cancer screening and detection of residual disease.	Image resolution needs to be improved.

Application of quantum dots in molecular and cellular imaging of the OSCC together *in vivo* and *in vitro* is gaining importance (Fixler et al. 2014, 602). They are nano- semiconductor crystals which luminesce through quantum confinement effects and have many advantages like size-tuneable emission, high luminescence, and large range of excitation spectra and are not easily affected by photo-bleaching (Bera et al. 2014, 2260). Moreover, manipulating the width and constitution of these dots allows a wide range of spectrum, from near ultraviolet to the near infrared. *In vivo* studies have used quantum dots linked to biomolecules in specific targeted therapies for treating oral carcinoma (Rosenthal et al. 2011, 10). It was found quantum dots having wavelengths of 700-900 nm in the near-infrared spectra have good tissue penetrating ability without cytotoxicity *in vivo* and therefore can be conjugated with monoclonal antibodies in targeted therapies in OSCC while those with emission wavelengths between 400-600 nm could be used for bio-imaging as they do not interfere with tissue auto-fluorescence (Yang et al. 2010, 864; Aswathy et al. 2010, 1417).

2.8. Nano-Based Ultrasensitive Biomarker Detection

Current research is focussed on new proteomic, genomic, and transcriptomic biomarkers for oral carcinoma. Molecular tumour biomarkers like the vascular endothelial growth factor (VEGF), tumour necrosis factor-alpha (TNF-α), EGFR, and interleukin 6 (IL 6) have been under investigation for early oral cancer diagnosis (Saxena et al. 2017, 90). However common estimation methods, including enzyme-linked immunosorbent assay (ELISA), Western Blot and polymerase chain reaction (PCR) have poor detection sensitivity (Li et al. 2018, 4807). Hence application of nanotechnology could enhance the sensitivity of these molecular bio-markers for oral carcinoma in low concentration.

3. Therapeutic Applications of Nanoparticle-Based Drug Delivery Systems in OSCC

OSCC is the commonest malignant neoplasm in the neck and head region and surgery and radiotherapy remain the mainstay of treatment. However advanced oral cancer treatment needs adjuvant chemotherapy (CT). It has been seen that CT greatly improves overall survival with reduction in recurrence. Cisplatin and 5-Fluorouracil are the most frequently used chemotherapeutic drugs. Molecular-targeted therapy, gene therapy, photo-dynamic therapy and immune-therapy have also been tried with limited efficacy (Zhu et al. 2009, 1). To enhance the efficacy and increase the safety of CT, nanotechnology-based platforms are the emergent cancer therapeutic regimens.

Nanoparticle (NP) platforms showed better drug carrying capabilities with site specific concentration of the therapeutic agents in malignant cells. Many pre-clinical studies in NP based chemo-therapeutic platforms revealed higher drug solubility, increased drug circulation times, and efficacy in comparison to conventional therapeutic regimens. Though there are NP based platforms available for treating ovarian and breast carcinoma, none is available for OSCC (Haley et al. 2008, 57). Nanomedicine systems can be versatile in their design to overcome biologic barriers like sequestration from phagocytic cells and concentrate in malignant tumours with increased permeability and retention (Xu et al. 2014, 6198). There are three generations of nanoparticle-based systems and their important features are summarized below:

Table 2. Principal features of nanoparticles of the three generations and the findings from research on oral squamous cell carcinoma (Ding et al. 2015)

FIRST GENERATION	SECOND GENERATION	THIRD GENERATION
➢ Passive extravasation in malignant tumours due to enhanced permeability and retention. ➢ Efficacy against primaries. ➢ No effect on regional lymph node metastasis.	➢ Active targeting for enhanced accumulation ➢ Controlled release of active agents ➢ Action against primary tumour. ➢ Overcomes chemoresistance.	➢ Migration towards and adhesion to tumour endothelium and local release of nanoparticles. ➢ Effective against distant metastasis ➢ Overcomes chemoresistance.

Summary of principal features of nanoparticles of first, second, and third generation and findings from preclinical or clinical studies in OSCC (first and second generation).

When the drug reaches the cell/tissue of interest (malignant cells) by using site specific ligands and the receptors at the target site by attaching the ligands to the nanoparticles, it is called active targeting (Pirollo et al. 2008, 552). Ligands are selected in a manner that they are concentrated on the malignant tumour cells and not the normal cells. Antibodies, nucleic acids, carbohydrates, vitamins, peptides, etc. have been used for attaching to nanoparticles. On attachment with the ligands, the NPs have an easy access to the target cell surface and drug delivery is easy and therapeutic response is achieved without adverse effects to the surroundings (Younga et al. 2014, 13383) (Figure 2).

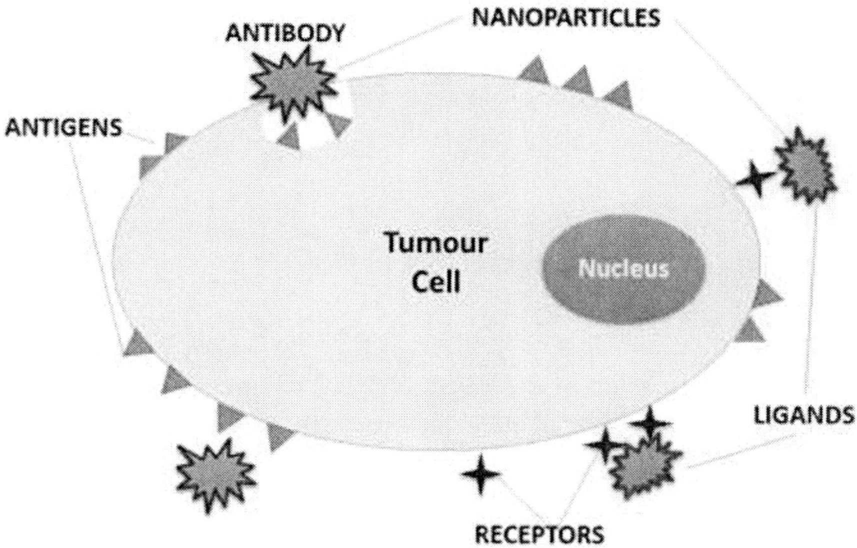

Figure 2. Association of NPs with receptors, ligands and the antigens.

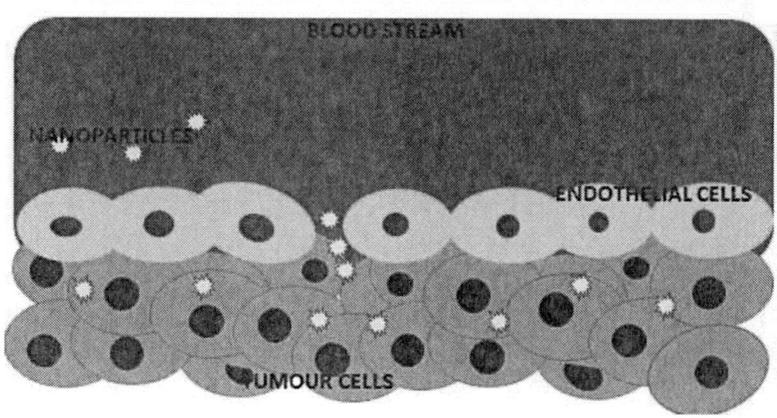

Figure 3. Enhanced permeability and retention based passive targeting of malignant cells by NPs based drug delivery systems.

The enhanced permeability and retention (EPR) effect is the basis of the passive drug transport used for targeting the malignant cells. Due to the lymphatic drainage normal cells does not accumulate the drugs but malignant cells have retention of the NPs based drugs and this preferential retention of the nanocarrier molecules is the fundamental principle for all NPs drug action in malignancies except hypovascular tumours, prostate and pancreatic cancer (Gabizon 1992, 891). The diagrammatic retention of passive targeting of malignant cells is shown below (Figure 3).

3.1. Nano-Based Chemoprevention in OSCC

Chemoprevention in OSCC uses therapeutic agents to prevent and supress the progression of dysplastic oral epithelial cells to malignancy. Flavonoids, carotenoids, curcumin, aloe vera, etc. have been promoted due to their anti-carcinogenic activity. But these herbal medicaments show poor solubility and bioavailability, thereby reducing their abilities. Hence NP-based chemo-preventive agents are being explored in trials to increase the efficacy (Gabizon 1992, 891; Sulfikkarali et al. 2013, 287).

NPs loaded with curcumin have been used in the therapy for OSCC therapy in a few studies and it was seen that polylactic co-glycolic acid (PLGA) NPs can exert a time and dose dependent reduction in the resistant tongue carcinoma cells. However, the normal epithelial cells and fibroblasts were unharmed (Afifi et al. 2013743; Chang et al. 2013, 1141). When treated with curcumin NPs, there was enhanced apoptosis, a hike in the reactive oxygen species (ROS) formation with down-regulation of the multiple drug resistance protein 1 (MDR1). When Curcumin was conjugated with Silica NPs, increase in cell uptake and cyto-toxicity in OSCC was seen than compared to free curcumin medicaments (Singh et al. 2014, 645). When the same curcumin conjugated silica NPs were used with LASERs there was increase in phototoxicity and cellular necrosis due to damage to cell membrane. When micro-emulsions with curcumin were used by Lin et al. together with low frequency ultrasonography, it was also found to be efficacious in comparison to free curcumin (Lin et al. 2002, 941).

Chitosan coated Polycaprolactone NPs with Curcumin was also employed in local therapy for OSCC and they caused apoptotic cell death of malignant tongue carcinoma cells in comparison to curcumin used singly (Mazzarino et al. 2013, 781).

Naringenin, a flavonoid which is derived from fruits has established anti-carcinogenic effects. In a hamster study by Sulfikkarali et al. (2013, 287), Naringenin-conjugated NPs treatment reduced the malignant tumour activity and decreased the dysplastic changes (Gavin et al. 2015, 1569). Gavin et al, used muco-adhesive chitosan coated nano-emulsions conjugated with genistein as buccal tablets which were found to be highly efficacious (Zhao et al. 2011, 534548). Li et al, further evaluated salvianolic acid B phospholipid complex-conjugated NPs in cell lines of oral potentially malignant cells and oral carcinoma cells and found that the proliferative activity of tumour cells was inhibited in both cell lines in comparison to free formulations of salvianolic acid B, a traditional Chinese medicament (Zhao et al. 2015, 9638).

3.2. Nanoparticle Based Chemotherapy

The novelty of nanotechnology lies in the site-specific action without any adverse reaction on the adjacent normal cells. CT is effective as an adjuvant therapy in advanced OSCC, but supportive evidence is lacking for its use as an induction therapy. The different nano-based platforms (Figure 4) and the advantages of nanotechnology in the delivery of drugs locally in oral cancer are shown (Figure 5). Hence many *in vitro* as well as *in vivo* studies have used NPs conjugated with chemotherapeutic agents like 5-flurouracil and molecular-targeted agents. 5-Fluorouracil-monomeric self-assembled nucleoside NPs was used by Zhao et al, (Zhao et al. 2015, 9638) *in vitro* and *in vivo* studies to determine their anti-cancer effect. Cyto-toxic effects on OSCC cells were seen in the long term than compared to 5-Fluorouracil given singly.

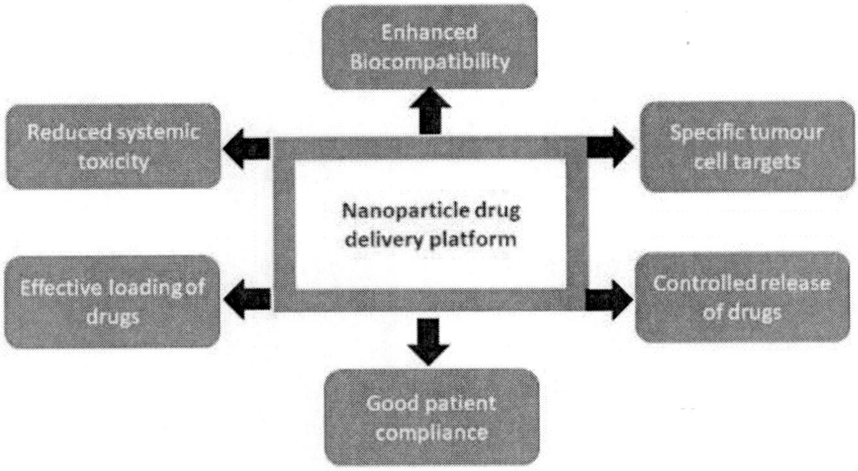

Figure 4. Advantages of using nano-platforms in drug delivery systems.

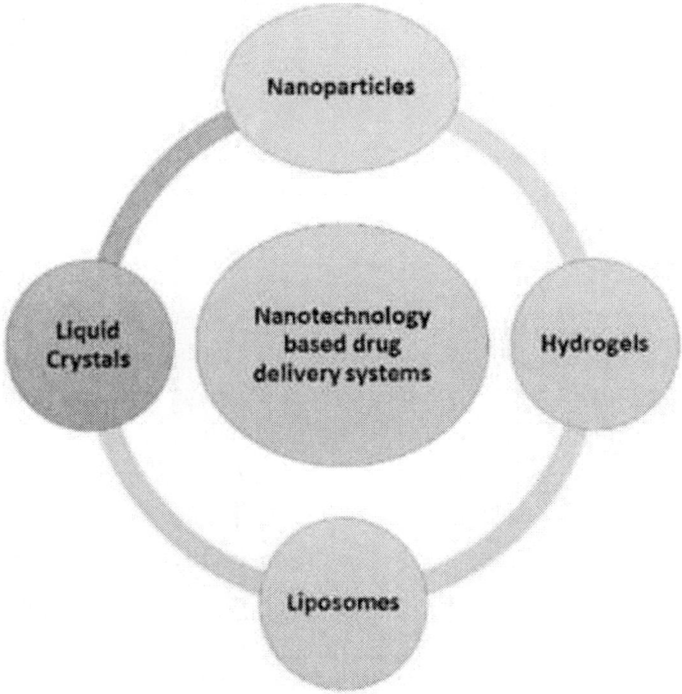

Figure 5. Different types of drug delivery systems based on nanotechnology used in oral cancer therapy.

Doxorubicin is an effective chemo-therapeutic agent but its clinical applications are hampered by cardiotoxicity. Therefore, a liposomal type of Doxorubicin was formulated to decrease the side effects and has been used as adjuvant chemotherapy in OSCC resulting in better results on primaries than on metastases (Koukourakis et al. 1999, 3512). Doxorubicin conjugated NPs have been formulated for OSCC therapy. The NPs drugs had better effect on OSCC cells in comparison to the non-conjugated and liposomal forms of Doxorubicin with enhanced apoptosis and DNA damage (Jain et al. 2012, 101).

Due to small size and the property of modifying their surface with antibodies, NPs were employed as theranostic agents, i.e., for diagnostic as well as therapeutic effects. Further because of their energy conversion capability, non-ionizing electromagnetic radiation from LASERs to heat, local induction of apoptosis is possible (Gabizon 1992, 891). Magnetic NPs have been also tried in research studies on humans for photo-thermal ablation of different tumours including OSCC (Satapathy et al. 2015, 4011).

Gold NPs are evolving for local drug carrying systems and photo-thermal systems. Colloidal gold NPs are prepared by reducing gold which on exposure to near-infrared light liberate heat. The efficiency of these gold NPs singly or in conjunction with LASERs has been investigated in animal studies (Afifi et al. 2013, 743). Gold NPs were injected directly into the malignant lesions and substantial decline in tumour growth was seen when gold NPs were used along with LASERs than used singly.

Gold shell having iron-core NPs were prepared to delay the oxidative process and increase the magnetic ability (Afifi et al. 2013, 743). It was seen that malignant cells were destroyed preferentially due to mitochondria-induced autophagy but the normal epithelial cells were spared. It was shown by Wu et al. (2011, 4565) that the gold NPs with iron core had specific cyto-toxic action on the dysplastic and malignant cells due to release of ferric ions seen both *in vivo* as well as *in vitro*.

Silica-core NPs with a gold coating used with photothermal therapy was employed in the treatment of refractory OSCC. Melancon et al, (Melancon et al. 2011, 7600) used gold nano-shells having a paramagnetic iron-silica core bound to cetuximab, a monoclonal antibody and it was compared with and without using LASERS. It was found that when targeted NPs were used with LASERs they exhibited the maximum cytotoxic effect.

CONCLUSION

The applications of nanotechnology in oral squamous cell carcinoma are not only diagnostic but also therapeutic which could have a profound effect on oral cancer care. Though many of the nano-particle based platforms are in the pre-clinical stages, with a potential to replace the conventional extremely invasive oral cancer detection and treatment including sentinel lymph node biopsies, radiotherapy and chemotherapy. Discovery of malignant changes at the earliest and treatment planning especially with targeted therapy without adverse effects on normal surrounding tissues would go a long way in decreasing the mortality and the morbidity related to this dreaded disease, leading to reduction in the cancer burden.

REFERENCES

Afifi M. M, El Sheikh S. M, Abdelsalam M. M, Ramadan H, Omar T. A, El Tantawi M, Abdel-Razek, K. M, Mohamed M, 2013. "Therapeutic efficacy of plasmonic photothermal nanoparticles in hamster buccal pouch carcinoma." *Oral Surg Oral Med Oral Pathol Oral Radiol* 115: 743–751. doi: 10.1016/j.oooo.2012.11.020.

Ankri R, Ashkenazy A, Milstein Y, Brami Y, Olshinka A, Goldenberg-Cohen N, Popovtzer A., Fixler D., Hirshberg A. 2016. "Gold nanorods based air scanning electron microscopy and diffusion reflection imaging for mapping tumor margins in squamous cell carcinoma." *ACS Nano.* 10: 2349–2356. doi: 10.1021/acsnano.5b07114.

Arakeri G, Patil S. G, Aljabab A. S, Lin K. C, Merkx M. A. W, Gao S, Brenann, P. A. 2017. "Oral submucous fibrosis: an update on pathophysiology of malignant transformation." *J Oral Pathol Med.* 46: 413–417. doi: 10.3322/caac.20107.

Aswathy R. G, Yoshida Y, Maekawa T, Kumar D. S. 2010. "Near-infrared quantum dots for deep tissue imaging." *Anal Bioanal Chem.* 397: 1417–1435. doi: 10.1007/s00216-010-3643-6.

Bayer C. L, Wlodarczyk B. J, Finnell R. H, Emelianov S. Y. 2017. "Ultrasound-guided spectral photoacoustic imaging of hemoglobin oxygenation during development." *Biomed Opt Express.* 8: 757–763. doi: 10.1364/BOE.8.000757.

Benergossi J, Calixto G, Fonseca-Santos B, Aida K. L, de Cassia Negrini T, Duque C, Gremiao, M. P. D, Chorilli M. 2015. "Highlights in peptide nanoparticle carriers intended to oral diseases." *Curr Top Med Chem.* 2015, 15: 345–355.

Bera D, Qian L, Tseng T. K, Holloway P. H. 2010. "Quantum dots and their multimodal applications: a review." *Materials.* 3: 2260–2345. doi: 10.3390/ma3042260.

Brigger I, Dubernet C, Couvreur P. 2002. "Nanoparticles in cancer therapy and diagnosis." *Adv Drug Deliv Rev.* 54: 631–651. doi: 10.1016/j.addr.2012.09.006.

Calixto G, Bernegossi J, Fonseca-Santos B, Chorilli M. 2014. "Nanotechnology-based drug delivery systems for treatment of oral cancer: a review." *Int J Nanomed.* 9: 3719–3735. doi: 10.2147/IJN.S61670.

Chandran P, Sasidharan A, Ashokan A, Menon D, Nair S, Koyakutty M. 2011. "Highly biocompatible TiO(2): Gd(3)(+) nano-contrast agent with enhanced longitudinal relaxivity for targeted cancer imaging." *Nanoscale.* 3: 4150–4161. doi: 10.1039/C1NR10591D.

Chang P. Y, Peng S. F, Lee C. Y, Lu C. C, Tsai S. C, Shieh T. M, Wu T. S, Tu M. G, Chem M. Y, Yang J. S. 2013. "Curcumin-loaded nanoparticles induce apoptotic cell death through regulation of the function of MDR1 and reactive oxygen species in cisplatin-resistant

CAR human oral cancer cells." *Int J Oncol* 43: 1141–1150. doi: 10.3892/ijo.2013.2050.

Chen C, Florian K, Rajesh K, Max R, Christian K, Florian S, Michael S. 2015. "Recovering the superficial microvascular pattern via diffuse reflection imaging: phantom validation." *Biomed Eng Online.* 14: 87. doi: 10.1186/s12938-015-0081-x.

Chen H, Kou X, Yang Z, Ni W, Wang J. 2008. "Shape- and size-dependent refractive index sensitivity of gold nanoparticles." *Langmuir.* 24: 5233–5237. doi: 10.1021/la800305j.

Cheng W, Ping Y, Zhang Y, Chuang K. H, Liu Y. 2013. "Magnetic resonance imaging (MRI) contrast agents for tumor diagnosis." *J Healthc Eng.* 4: 23–45. url: https://www.hindawi.com/journals/jhe/2013/143865/abs/.

Ding Y, Shen S. Z, Sun H, Sun K, Liu F, Qi Y, Yan J. 2015. "Design and construction of polymerized-chitosan coated Fe3O4 magnetic nanoparticles and its application for hydrophobic drug delivery Mater." *Sci. Eng. C* 48: 487-498. doi: 10.1016/j.msec.2014.12.036.

El-Sayed I. H, Huang X, El-Sayed M. A. 2005. "Surface plasmon resonance scattering and absorption of anti-EGFR antibody conjugated gold nanoparticles in cancer diagnostics: applications in oral cancer." *Nano Lett.* 5: 829–834. doi: 10.1021/nl050074e.

Fixler D, Ankri R, Kaplan I, Novikov I, Hirshberg A. 2014. "Diffusion reflection: a novel method for detection of oral cancer." *J Dent Res.* 93: 602–606. doi: 10.1177/0022034514529973.

Gabizon A. A. 1992. "Selective tumor localization and improved therapeutic index of anthracyclines encapsulated in long-circulating liposomes." *Cancer Res.* 52: 891-896. url: http://cancerres.aacr journals.org/content/52/4/891.article-info.

Gavin A, Pham J. T, Wang D, Brownlow B, Elbayoumi T. A. 2015. "Layered nanoemulsions as mucoadhesive buccal systems for controlled delivery of oral cancer therapeutics." *Int J Nanomed* 10: 1569–1584. doi: 10.2147/IJN.S75474.

Green B, Tsiroyannis C, Brennan P. A. 2016. "Optical diagnostic systems for assessing head and neck lesions." *Oral Dis.* 22: 180–184. doi:10.1 111/odi.12398.

Guze K, Pawluk H. C, Short M, Zeng H, Lorch J, Norris C, Sonis S. 2015. "Pilot study: Raman spectroscopy in differentiating premalignant and malignant oral lesions from normal mucosa and benign lesions in humans." *Head Neck.* 37: 511–517. doi: 10.1002/hed.23629.

Haley B, E. Frenkel. 2008. "Nanoparticles for drug delivery in cancer treatment. Urologic Oncology: Seminars and Original Investigations." *Elsevier* 57-64. doi: 10.1016/j.urolonc.2007.03.015.

Harmsen S, Wall M. A, Huang R. M, Kircher M. F. 2017. "Cancer imaging using surface-enhanced resonance Raman scattering nanoparticles." *Nat Protoc.* 12: 1400–1414. doi: 10.1038/nprot.2017.0 31.

Hinni M. L, Zarka M. A, Hoxworth J. M. 2013. "Margin mapping in transoral surgery for head and neck cancer." *Laryngoscope.* 123: 1190–1198. doi: 10.1002/lary.23900.

Hou C, Galvan D. D, Meng G, Yu Q. 2017. "Long-range surface plasmon resonance and surface-enhanced Raman scattering on X-shaped gold plasmonic nanohole arrays." *Phys Chem Chem Phys.* 19: 24126–24134. doi: 10.1039/C7CP04564F.

Jain S, Hirst D. G, O'Sullivan J. M. 2012. "Gold nanoparticles as novel agents for cancer therapy." *Br J Radiol* 85: 101–113. doi: 10.1259/b jr/59448833.

Jayanthi J. L, Nisha G. U, Manju S, Philip E. K, Jeemon P, Baiju K. V, Beena V. T, Subhash N. 2011. "Diffuse reflectance spectroscopy: diagnostic accuracy of a non-invasive screening technique for early detection of malignant changes in the oral cavity." *BMJ Open.* 1: e000071. doi: 10.1136/bmjopen-2011-000071.

Jemal A, Bray F, Center M. M, Ferlay J, Ward E, Forman D. 2011. "Global cancer statistics." *CA Cancer J Clin.* 61: 69–90. doi: 10.3322/caac.20107.

Jiang Y, Pu K. 2017. "Advanced photoacoustic imaging applications of near-infrared absorbing organic nanoparticles." *Small.* 13: 1700710. doi: 10.1002/smll.201700710.

Kah J. C, Kho K. W, Lee C. G, James C, Sheppard R, Shen Z. X, Soo K. C, Olivo M. C. 2007. "Early diagnosis of oral cancer based on the surface plasmon resonance of gold nanoparticles." *Int J Nanomed.* 2: 785–798. url: https://www.dovepress.com/articles.php?article_id=729.

Kang J. W, So PTC, Dasari R. R, Lim D. K. 2015. "High resolution live cell Raman imaging using subcellular organelle-targeting SERS-sensitive gold nanoparticles with highly narrow intra-nanogap." *Nano Lett.* 15: 1766–1772. doi: 10.1021/nl504444w.

Kim C. S, Wilder-Smith P, Ahn Y. C, Liaw L. H, Chen Z, Kwon Y. J. 2009. "Enhanced detection of early-stage oral cancer in vivo by optical coherence tomography using multimodal delivery of gold nanoparticles." *J Biomed Opt.* 14: 034008. doi: 10.1117/1.3130323.

Koukourakis M. I, Koukouraki S, Giatromanolaki A, Archimandritis S. C, Skarlatos J, Beroukas K, Bizakis J. G, Ritalis G., Karkavitsas N., Helidonis E. S. 1999. "Liposomal doxorubicin and conventionally fractionated radiotherapy in the treatment of locally advanced non-small-cell lung cancer and head and neck cancer." *J Clin Oncol* 17: 3512–3521. url: http://citeseerx.ist.psu.edu/viewdoc/download?doi=10.1.1.961.8862&rep=rep1&type=pdf.

Lin H. Y., Thomas J. L., Chen H. W., Shen C. M., Yang W. J., Lee M. H, 2002. "In vitro suppression of oral squamous cell carcinoma growth by ultrasound-mediated delivery of curcumin micro emulsions." *Int J Nanomed* 7: 941. doi: 10.2147/IJN.S28510.

Li X, Wei L, Pan L, Yi Z, Wang X, Ye Z, Xiao L., Li H. W., Wang J. 2018. "Homogeneous immunosorbent assay based on single-particle enumeration using up-conversion nanoparticles for the sensitive detection of cancer biomarkers." *Anal Chem.* 90: 4807–4814. doi: 10.1021/acs.analchem.8b00251.

Liang S, Li C, Zhang C, Chen Y, Xu L, Bao C, Wang X, Liu G, Zhang F, Cui D. 2015. "CD44v6 monoclonal antibody-conjugated gold nanostars for targeted photoacoustic imaging and plasmonic photothermal therapy of gastric cancer stem-like cells." *Theranostics.* 5: 970–984. doi: 10.7150/thno.11632.

Liu D, Zhao X, Zeng X, Dan H, Chen Q. 2016. "Non-invasive techniques for detection and diagnosis of oral potentially malignant disorders." *Tohoku J Exp Med.* 238: 165–177. doi: 10.1620/tjem.238.165.

Liu Q, Wang J, Wang B, Li Z, Huang H, Li C, Yu X, Chu P. K. 2014. "Paper-based plasmonic platform for sensitive, noninvasive, and rapid cancer screening." *Biosens Bioelectron.* 54: 128–134. doi: 10.1016/j.b ios.2013.10.067.

Liu R, Zhao J, Han G, Zhao T, Zhang R, Liu B, Liu Z, Zhang C, Yang L, Zhang Z. 2017. "Click-functionalized SERS nanoprobes with improved labeling efficiency and capability for cancer cell imaging." *ACS Appl Mater Interfaces.* 9: 38222–38229. doi:10.1021/acsam i.7b1 0409.

Luke G. P, Myers J. N, Emelianov S. Y, Sokolov K. V. 2014. "Sentinel lymph node biopsy revisited: ultrasound-guided photoacoustic detection of micrometastases using molecularly targeted plasmonic nanosensors." *Cancer Res.* 74: 5397–5408. doi: 10.1158/0008-547 2.CAN-14-0796.

Mazzarino L, Loch-Neckel G, Bubniak L. D. S, Mazzucco S, Santos-Silva M. C, Borsali R, Elenara L. S. 2015. "Curcumin-loaded chitosan-coated nanoparticles as a new approach for the local treatment of oral cavity cancer." *J Nanosci Nanotechnol* 15: 781–791. doi: 10.1166/ jnn.2015.9189.

Melancon M. P, Lu W, Zhong M, Zhou M, Liang G, Elliott A. M, Hazle J. D, Myers J. N, Li C, Stafford R. J. 2011. "Targeted multifunctional gold-based nano shells for magnetic resonance-guided laser ablation of head and neck cancer." *Biomaterials* 32: 7600–7608. doi: 10.1016/j. biomaterials.2011.06.039.

Ng J. H, Iyer N. G, Tan M. H, Edgren G. 2017. "Changing epidemiology of oral squamous cell carcinoma of the tongue: a global study." *Head Neck.* 39: 297–304. doi: 10.1002/hed.24589.

Oldenburg A. L, Hansen M. N, Zweifel D. A, Wei A, Boppart S. A. 2006. "Plasmon-resonant gold nanorods as low backscattering albedo contrast agents for optical coherence tomography." *Opt Express.* 14: 6724–6738. doi: 10.1364/OE.14.006724.

Pirollo K. F, Chang E. H. 2008. "Does a targeting ligand influence nanoparticle tumor localization or uptake?" *Trends Biotechnol.* 26: 552-558. doi: 10.1016/j.tibtech.2008.06.007.

Rosenthal S. J, Chang J. C, Kovtun O, McBride J. R, Tomlinson I. D. 2011. "Biocompatible quantum dots for biological applications." *Chem Biol.* 18: 10–24. doi: 10.1016/j.oraloncology.2010.09.009.

Sarrion Perez M. G, Bagan J. V, Jimenez Y, Margaix M, Marzal C. 2015. "Utility of imaging techniques in the diagnosis of oral cancer." *J Craniomaxillofac Surg.* 43: 1880–1894. doi: 10.1016/j.jcms.2015.07.0 37.

Satapathy S. R, Siddharth S, Das D, Nayak A, Kundu C. N. 2015. "Enhancement of cytotoxicity and inhibition of angiogenesis in oral cancer stem cells by a hybrid nanoparticle of bioactive quinacrine and silver: implication of base excision repair cascade." *Mol Pharm* 12: 4011–4025. doi: 10.1021/acs.molpharmaceut.5b00461.

Saxena S, Sankhla B, Sundaragiri K. S, Bhargava A. 2017. "A review of salivary biomarker: a tool for early oral cancer diagnosis." *Adv Biomed Res.* 6: 90. doi: 10.4103/2277-9175.211801.

Shanavas A, Sasidharan S, Bahadur D, Srivastava R. 2017. "Magnetic core-shell hybrid nanoparticles for receptor targeted anti-cancer therapy and magnetic resonance imaging." *J Colloid Interface Sci.* 486: 112–120. doi: 10.1016/j.jcis.2016.09.060.

Siegel R. L, Miller K. D, Jemal A. 2016. "Cancer statistics." *CA Cancer J Clin.* 66: 7–30. doi: 10.3322/caac.21332.

Singh S. P, Sharma M, Gupta P. K. 2014. "Enhancement of phototoxicity of curcumin in human oral cancer cells using silica nanoparticles as delivery vehicle." *Lasers Med Sci.* 29: 645–652. doi: 10.1007/s10103-013-1357-7.

Sokolov K, Follen M, Aaron J, Pavlova I, Malpica A, Lotan R, Richards-Kortum R. 2003. "Real-time vital optical imaging of precancer using anti-epidermal growth factor receptor antibodies conjugated to gold nanoparticles." *Cancer Res.* 63: 1999–2004. url: http://cancerres.aacr journals.org/content/63/9/1999.article-info.

Sulfikkarali N, Krishnakumar N, Manoharan S, Nirmal R. M. 2013. "Chemopreventive efficacy of naringenin-loaded nanoparticles in 7, 12-dimethylbenz (a) anthracene induced experimental oral carcinogenesis." *Pathol Oncol Res* 19: 287–296. doi: 10.1007/s12253-012-9581-1.

Tanaka T, Ishigamori R. 2011. "Understanding carcinogenesis for fighting oral cancer." *J Oncol.* 2011: 603740. doi: 10.1155/2011/603740.

Tasche K. K, Buchakjian M. R, Pagedar N. A, Sperry S. M. 2017. "Definition of "Close Margin" in oral cancer surgery and association of margin distance with local recurrence rate." *JAMA Otolaryngol Head Neck Surg.* 143: 1166–1172. doi: 10.1001/jamaoto.2017.0548.

Torre L. A, Bray F, Siegel R. L, Ferlay J, Lortet-Tieulent J, Jemal A. 2015. "Global cancer statistics." *CA Cancer J Clin.* 65: 87–108. doi.org/10.3322/caac.21262.

Wang J. H, Wang B, Liu Q, Li Q, Huang H, Song L, Sun T. Y, Wang H, Yu X. F, Li C, Chu P. K. 2013. "Bimodal optical diagnostics of oral cancer based on rose bengal conjugated gold nano rod platform." *Biomaterials.* 34: 4274–4283. doi: 10.1016/j.biomaterials.2013.02.012.

Warnakulasuriya S. 2009. "Global epidemiology of oral and oropharyngeal cancer." *Oral Oncol.* 45: 309-316. doi: 10.1016/j.oraloncology.2008.06.002.

Wu Y. N, Yang L. X, Shi X. Y, Li I. C, Biazik J. M, Ratinac K. R, Chen D. H, Thordarson P, Shieh D. B, Braet F. 2011. "The selective growth inhibition of oral cancer by iron core-gold shell nanoparticles through mitochondria- mediated autophagy." *Biomaterials* 32: 4565–4573. doi: 10.1016/j.biomaterials.2011.03.006.

Xiao-Jie C, Zhang X, Qi Liu, Gang Z. 2018. "Nanotechnology: a promising method for oral cancer detection and diagnosis." *Journal of Nanobiotechnology* 16: 52. doi: 10.1186/s12951-018-0378-6.

Xu C, Chen F, Valdovinos H. F, Jiang D, Goel S, Yu B, Sun H, Barnhart T. E, Moon J. J, Cai W. 2018. "Bacteria-like mesoporous silica-coated gold nanorods for positron emission tomography and photoacoustic imaging-guided chemo-photothermal combined therapy." *Biomaterials.* 165: 56–65. doi: 10.1016/j.biomaterials.2018.02.043.

Xu Y, Baiu D. C, Sherwood J. A, Mc. Elreath M. R, Qin Y, Lackey K. H, Otto M, Bao Y. 2014. "Linker-free conjugation and specific cell targeting of antibody functionalized iron-oxide nanoparticles." *J. Mater. Chem. B* 2: 6198-6206. doi: 10.1039/C4TB00840E.

Yan B, Li B, Wen Z, Luo X, Xue L, Li L. 2015. "Label-free blood serum detection by using surface-enhanced Raman spectroscopy and support vector machine for the preoperative diagnosis of parotid gland tumors." *BMC Cancer.* 15: 650. doi: 10.1186/s12885-015-1653-7.

Yang K, Cao Y. A, Shi C, Li Z. G, Zhang F. J, Yang J, Zhao C. 2010. "Quantum dot-based visual in vivo imaging for oral squamous cell carcinoma in mice." *Oral Oncol.* 46: 864–868. doi: 10.1016/j.oraloncology.2010.09.009.

Youngá Y. J. 2014. "Advances in targeting strategies for nanoparticles in cancer imaging and therapy." *Nanoscale* 6: 13383-13390. doi: 10.1039/c4nr04334k.

Zhang M, Kim H. S, Jin T, Yi A, Moon W. K. 2016. "Ultrasound-guided photoacoustic imaging for the selective detection of EGFR-expressing breast cancer and lymph node metastases." *Biomed Opt Express.* 7: 1920–1931. doi: 10.1364/BOE.7.001920.

Zhao H, Feng H, Liu D, Liu J, Ji N, Chen F, Luo X, Zhou Y, Dan H, Zeng X, Li X, Sun C, Meng J, Ju X, Zhou M, Yang H, Li L, Liang X, Chu L, Jiang L, He Y, Chen Q. 2015. "Self-assembling monomeric nucleoside molecular nanoparticles loaded with 5-FU enhancing therapeutic efficacy against oral cancer." *ACS Nano* 9: 9638–9651. doi: 10.1021/acsnano.5b04520.

Zhao Y, Guo Y, Gu X. 2011. "Salvianolic acid B, a potential chemopreventive agent, for head and neck squamous cell cancer." *J Oncol* 2011: 534548. doi: 10.1155/2011/534548.

Zhu, L., Ma, J., Jia, N., Zhao, Y., Shen, H. 2009. "Chitosan-coated magnetic nanoparticles as carriers of 5-fluorouracil: preparation, characterization and cytotoxicity studies." *Colloids Surf. B* 68: 1–6. doi: 10.1016/j.colsurfb.2008.07.020.

In: Nanoparticles
Editors: A. K. Samantara, S. Ratha
ISBN: 978-1-53616-596-8

Chapter 6

NANOPARTICLES AND ITS CONJUGATES APPLICATION IN DENTISTRY

Lora Mishra[1,*], Satyaranjan Misra[2] and Gunjan Srivastav[3]

[1]Department of Conservative Dentistry and Endontics, Institute of Dental Sciences, Siksha 'O' Anusandhan University, Bhubaneswar, Odisha, India

[2]Department of Oral Medicine and Radiology, Institute of Dental Sciences, Siksha 'O' Anusandhan University, Bhubaneswar, Odisha, India

[3]Department of Prosthodontics, Institute of Dental Sciences, Siksha'O'Anusandhan University, Bhubaneswar, Odisha, India

ABSTRACT

The mouth is the gateway to the overall health of the human being. The mouth comprises of hard tissue and soft tissue structures. The main purpose of these structures is to aid in mastication, speech, swallowing etc. There is no tissue as hard as dental enamel in the human body. Tooth

---

* Corresponding Author's Email: loramishra@soa.ac.in.

enamel, once lost, cannot be replaced back. But with the discovery of nanoparticles, this dream has become reality. Many researchers have been working to create appropriate replaceable structures that would mimic these biological structures, both functionally and aesthetically. Nanoparticles have been playing a major role in the diagnostic and therapeutic arena because of their size. In the context of being used as fillers to enhance mechanical properties of dental materials, as active media for local drug delivery systems, their application is widespread. They can also be manufactured in large scale and can be cost effective.

Keywords: biocompatibility, caries, dentistry, fillers, nanoparticles

1. INTRODUCTION

Dentistry depends on diagnosis, therapeutics and dental materials. Diagnosis and therapeutics aid in maintaining oral health and also give insight to overall systemic health of the patient. Dental material is a very important aspect of dentistry. There has been a constant change and evolution in this field of medical sciences, especially dental science. This branch of dentistry deals with the fabrication, invention and discovery of those materials which would mimic the natural tooth structure. The tooth structure can be lost due to caries, trauma, deleterious and parafunctional habits. Furthermore, it is subject to constant wear and tear. The dental material should be capable of tolerating such dynamic changes in the mouth. Nanotechnology can provide a formidable and long term solution to present demand of dentistry. It has a plethora of uses which includes dental diagnosis, dental material and therapy for oro-dental diseases. It metamorphosed the dental science by enhancing the various physico-mechanical properties of dental materials, providing newer diagnostic methods, and nanoparticle-based delivery systems (AlKahtani 2018, 107).

2. Application of Nanotechnology in Dentistry

2.1. Application in Diagnosis

The utility of nano-technology in dentistry encompasses 3 broad areas, as depicted in Figure 1. (AlKahtani 2018, 107).

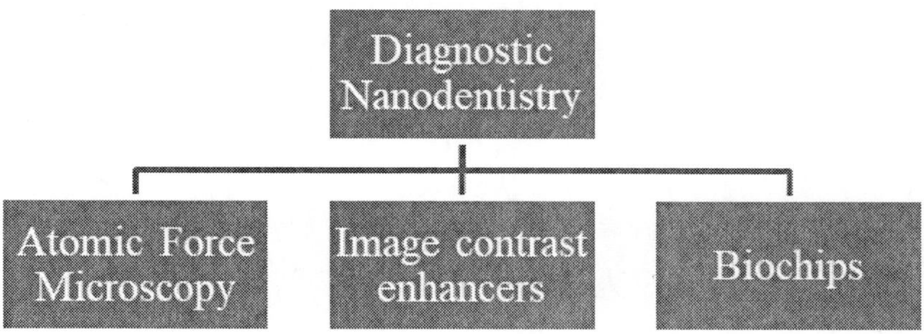

Figure 1. Illustrating the broad area of dentistry and medicine in which their application is vital. Nanoparticles are utilised in the area of multiple diagnostic devices. Their inclusion in advanced diagnostic aids has led to breakthrough discoveries in the visualisation of human tissue in a non-invasive way.

2.2. Dental Health

Interception and early disease detection are crucial for sustaining good oral health. The development of miniature, flexible, and wireless biosensors will provide the opportunity to utilize the oral cavity as a region to gather information on vital physiological, metabolic and toxicological signatures. The various applications are listed in Figure 2.

Nanoparticles are manufactured by using any of the following approaches: top down, bottom up, or the molecular self-assembly approach. The replacement of micro-sized particles with nano-sized ones has the capacity to transform the biosensor into a nano-biosensor, with the benefit of having rapid identification in targeted biological tissues at an ultra-low molecular level (Jorio 2016). AFM provides real time images of different biofilms which generally adhere to the tooth structure. This enables us to understand the interaction of these complex microorganism networks with tooth structure and helps in the prevention and/or treatment of biofilm dependent diseases like dental caries.

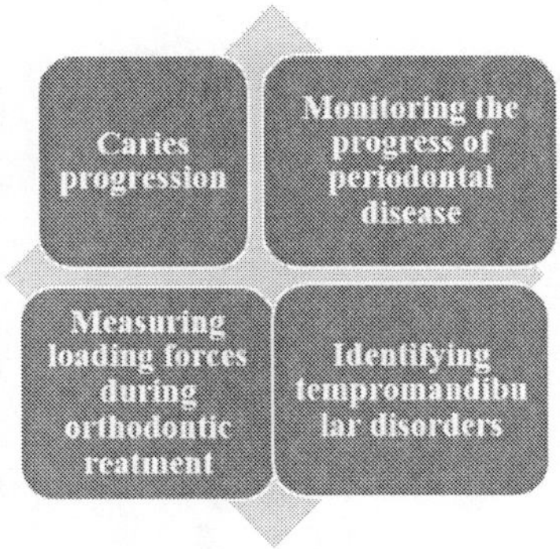

Figure 2. Illustrating the various applications of nanoparticles.

2.3. Oral Cancer

CT scans, magnetic resonance imaging and ultrasounds are routinely used for diagnosing oral cancers. These techniques can help us identify the site, size and spread of tumour cells. The only limitation these techniques have is that they are not able to differentiate between benign and malignant/cancerous tumours. Early cancer lesions, which are smaller than 5 mm are also not visualised by these imaging techniques (Popovtzer 2008, 4593). Image contrast enhancers in the form nanoparticles add substantial value to these imaging techniques (Figure 3).

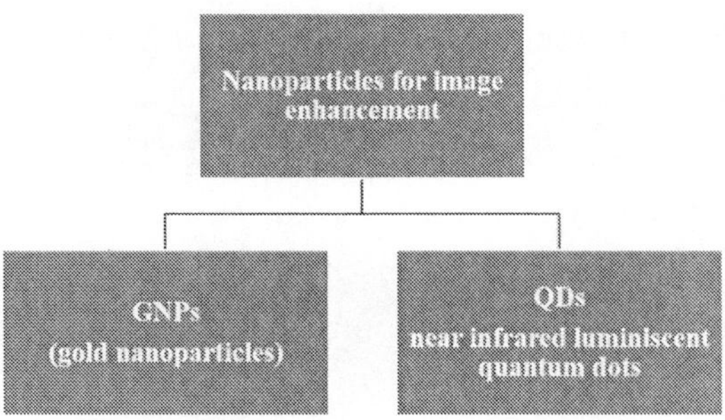

Figure 3. Nanoparticles' based image contrasting agents.

Gold, being a noble metal, exhibits a strong X-ray absorption property, which enables it for being used as a contrast agent in the form of gold nano-particles (GNPs). To functionalize it in the form of GNPs, ligands like polyethylene glycol have to be used, so that both the stability and persistence of the molecules (gold) are maintained in the blood circulation, thereby enhancing accumulation concentration in the malignant tumour tissue. Such behaviour is of great help when it comes to imaging cancer affected tissues (Neel 2015, 6371).

Besides GNPs, quantum dots (QDs) are nanometer-scale semi-conductor crystals, which act as inorganic fluorophores when exposed to a light energy resonating with their excitation wavelength. Like GNPs, they may also be conjugated with different biomolecules. Thus, the QDs, when functionalized, can be used as selective luminescent probes that can effectively bind with specificity and sensitivity to a variety of targets. Yang et al., in his research, utilized peptides which could penetrate cells when conjugated with NIR QDs, for the diagnosis of oral cancer (Neel 2015, 6371).

2.4. Biochips and Salivary Biomarkers

Saliva has been routinely used by dentists and oral biologists to evaluate caries risk assessment of an individual. Streptococcus mutans and lactobacillus culture courts gives lot of information about the caries exposure of a patient. Any variation in salivary level of estrogen, testosterone, progesterone and electrolytes, also gives clues about female reproductive health and overall health of an individual. At present, saliva based nano chip has been developed for acute myocardial infarction and for cytological diagnosis of oral cancers, as has been discussed below. Recently, non-invasive exfoliative cytology, Oral CDx® Brush Test (OralScan Laboratories, Suffern, NY), has been widely promoted for the screening of oral cancer. This particular method utilizes the quantitative cyto-morphometry principle and DNA aneuploidy computer-assisted analysis.

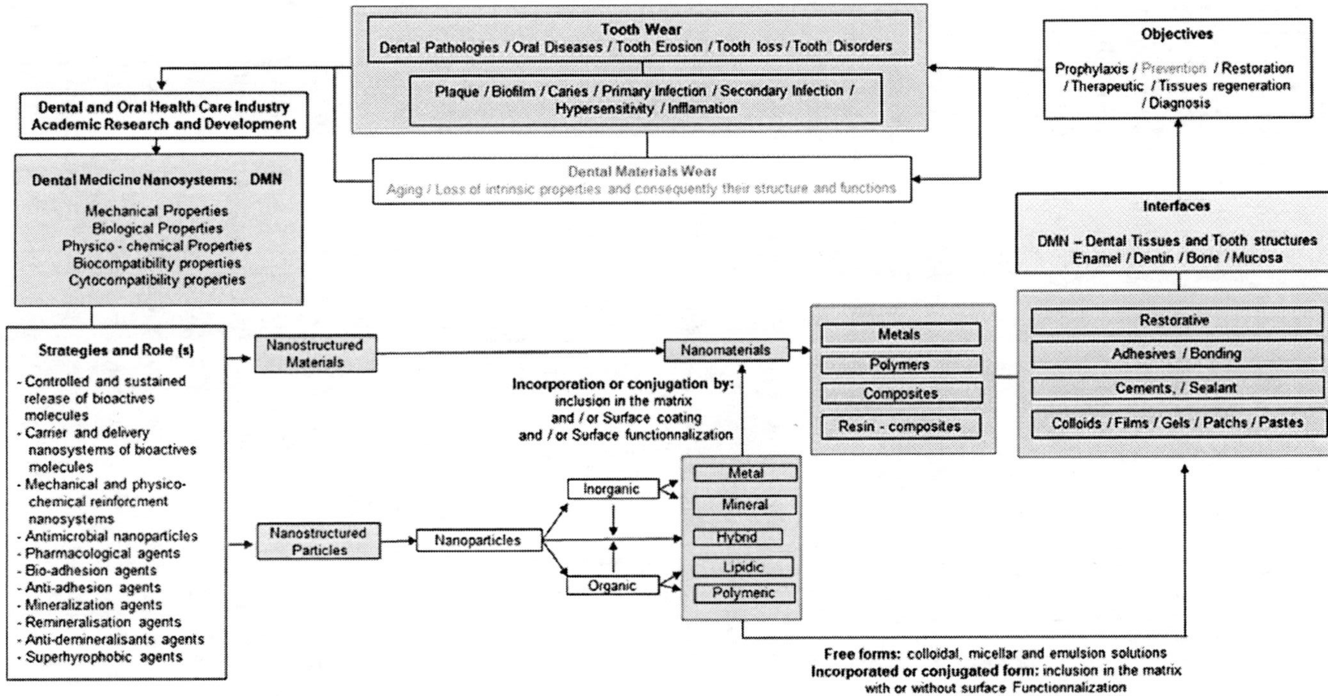

Figure 4. Nano particles in Therapeutics. Illustration of Dental Medicine Nanosystems design and the strategies of their use for preventive, therapeutic, restoration, tissue regeneration and their combination. (Lboutounne 2017, 145).

2.5. Dental/Prophylactic Prevention Treatments

Recently, lots of emphasis is done on preventive therapy than on treatment in the context of management of dental diseases. Dental diseases are classified into carious lesion and non-carious lesion. Caries is a microbiological disease, which leads to the destruction of tooth structure. Non-carious lesion, which occurs due to parafunctional or deleterious habits, could cause unnatural wearing of tooth structure. It is believed that the formation of the components of tooth structure is an irreversible procedure, hence strategies are being adopted to either slow or reverse the caries procedure or make dental materials tooth like. Numerous researches have been carried out to incorporate these nano particles in dentistry, which will not only protect the tooth from carious attack but also impart a therapeutic effect by regeneration of lost tissues. Nanoparticles, depending on their source, are classified into inorganic, organic and hybrid. Inorganic particles like silver, zirconium are added to dental materials to enhance the physical properties of the material. Recently, chitosan derivative from shells of crustaceans has also been used in disinfecting and irrigating the solution, which is being used during root canal treatment. There are plethora of scopes for nanoparticles in dentistry and many academicians and researchers are working towards exploring the same (Figure 5).

Synthesis of nanotechnology basically involves two major approaches such as top down and bottom up growth process, to obtain tinier particles at nanoscale, for improving dental materials with complex assembly. Processing of materials in the solid state is done in the top-down approach, as seen in milling, machining and lithography. Chemical vapour deposition (CVD), wet and plasma etching, monolithic processing are methods which utilize fabrication of functional structures at nano and micro scales. The manufacturing of medical implants and stents uses CVD technology to achieve biocompatibility. When materials are fabricated by harvesting of atomic elements to form bulk structures, the approach is referred to as the "bottom-up" approach. Nature shows the best example of bottom-up approach like cell, tissue or organ repair and synthesis of proteins (Khursh 2015, 717).

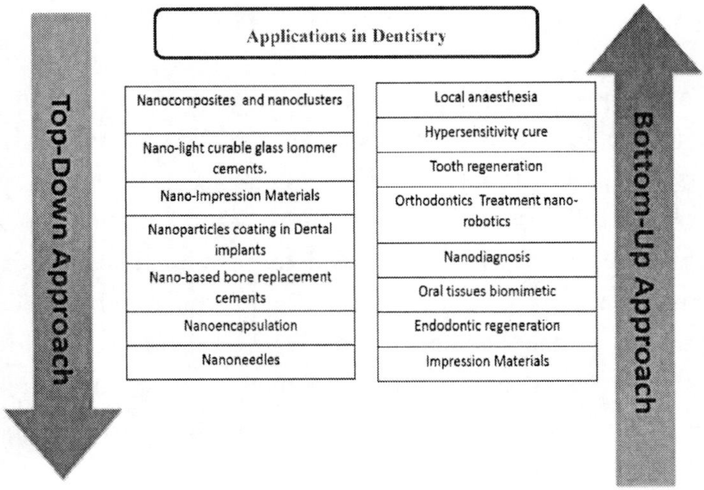

Figure 5. Breakthrough approaches of nanotechnology applications in dentistry.

2.6. Dental Biomaterials

Nanoparticles were incorporated in materials to utilize their enormous potential for use in different medical and dental applications. Nanoparticles comprise of groups of atoms having a size range of 1–100 nm. The most promising of all nanoparticles are the metallic ones, which have anti-bacterial effects. Also, because of their larger surface are to volume ratios, they have been attracting considerable attention from researchers due to the challenges faced because of microbial resistance against metal ions, antibacterial drugs and the resurgence of resistant strains. Metallic nanoparticles could be used as efficacious growth inhibitors for different micro-organisms and hence can be used in various medical devices for varieties of applications. Nanotechnology encompasses the use of elemental nanoparticles as the active anti-bacterial substances in dental materials (Hamouda 2012, 143). Silver nanoparticles, the most commonly used NPs, are used in different products in various forms, while carbon and titaniun oxide (TiO_2) have also been used (RA 2012). The applications in dentistry can either provide therapeutic, antimicrobial or can be simply used to reinforce the existing dental material (Figure 6).

Table 3. Properties of nanoparticles

Nanoparticles	Compressive strength, Malleability, ductility	Physical property	Chemical property
Carbon nanotubes	Carbon nanotubes can offer tensile strength because of the hexagonal arrangement, yet it has the malleability of rubber, high tensile ductility (8–13%), and good mechanical strength.	Surface area is large, ultra-light-weight, heat stability, high strength, and less dense.	Heat transmission efficiency. Strong bond between carbons atoms make this material quite stable; the carbon atoms in nanotubes are arranged in hexagonal rings.
Graphene	Graphene is transparent, flexible (high malleability and ductility) and highly stable.	The unique structure gives rise to a high planar surface area, superior mechanical strength, electronic properties are remarkable and alluring optical characteristics.	Single atom thick carbon sheets of honeycomb lattice oriented in a two-dimensional (2D) fashion make up the graphene structure. Due to the structure, graphene has acquired a number of unique and exceptional physico-chemical characters.
Hydroxy apatite (HAp)		Greater surface area, hexagonal structure.	It is a calcium phosphate. It is quite stable when compared to other calcium phosphates.
Zirconia	The ductile, soft and malleable matter which provides great resistance to corrosion.	Zirconium nanoparticles are lighter and less susceptible to embrittlement by hydrogen.	Available in the form of nanodots, Nano fluids nanocrystals with the white surface area. Provide great resistance to corrosion by acids, alkalis, salt water and other agents.

Table 3. (Continued)

Nanoparticles	Compressive strength, Malleability, ductility	Physical property	Chemical property
Silica	Compressive strength–1600 MPa with minimal ductility and significant hardness.	Two types based on their structure – P-type and S-type. P-type is characterized by numerous Nano pores whereas S-type is having smaller surface area. P-type nano silica is having comparatively higher UV reflectivity.	Chemical Composition Silica -46.83% Oxygen 53.33% Molar mass 59.96g/mol Density- 2.4g/cm3
Titania	Have a compressive strength of about 3675 MPa with null ductility, quite hard and an elasticity limit of 367.5 MPa.	Found as nanocrystals or nano drops having large surface area, exhibit magnetic properties.	Chemical Composition Titania- 59.3% Oxygen- 40.55% Insoluble in water & organic solvent
Silver	Silver nanoparticles have high ductility and malleability. They are also good conductors.	Small size, the surface area is large, having exceptional optical, electrical and thermal conductivity.	Chemically very stable having catalytic activity, unique surface chemistry which helps them better act as an antimicrobial agent.

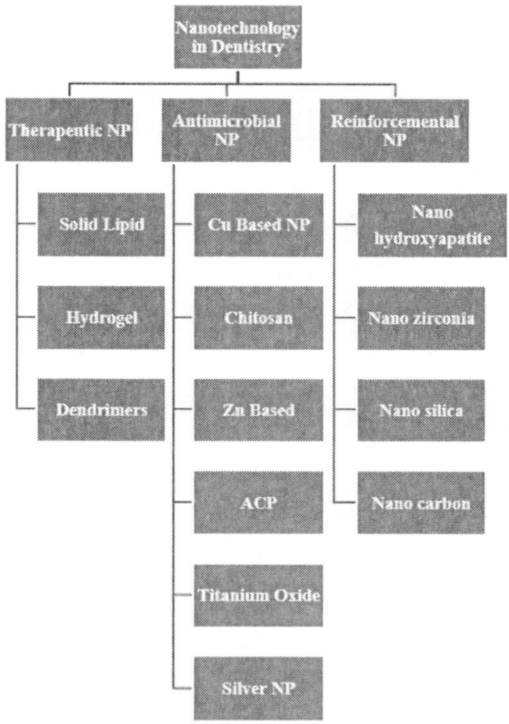

Figure 6. Dental application of nanoparticles.

3. Nanoparticle

3.1. Inorganic Nanoparticles

3.1.1. Carbon Nanotubes

Carbon nanotubes (CNTs) are garnering a lot of attention due to their unique physical properties and different applications (Figure 7). Recent studies have shown that CNTs can be used as biomedical materials owing to their unique properties, (Akasaka 2009, 179); some of which are listed below.

- Improve the strength of composite materials and implants
- Increase cell adhesion and proliferation

- Effect nucleation of hydroxyapatite
- Provide protection against bacteria

CNTs are now being utilized in various applications in dentistry, particularly in restorative and reparative dental tissue procedures. CNT have great thermal, mechanical and electric properties with easy functionalization and biocompatibility. In oral regenerative medication, bone reconstruction is a vital requirement for functional rehabilitation of the stomatognathic system. Autologous bone still represents the most popular graft material for bone reconstruction, but the small quantities of bone available in donor regions, together with the excessive fees of surgeries, are important elements that avoid the choice of this technique. CNTs, alone or combined with biopolymers, therefore, have promise for being used as potential biomaterials for the restoration of bone defects. Indeed, current evidence demonstrates CNT to be a feasible fabric, which could generate the formation of bone in tooth (Martins-Júnior 2013, 575).

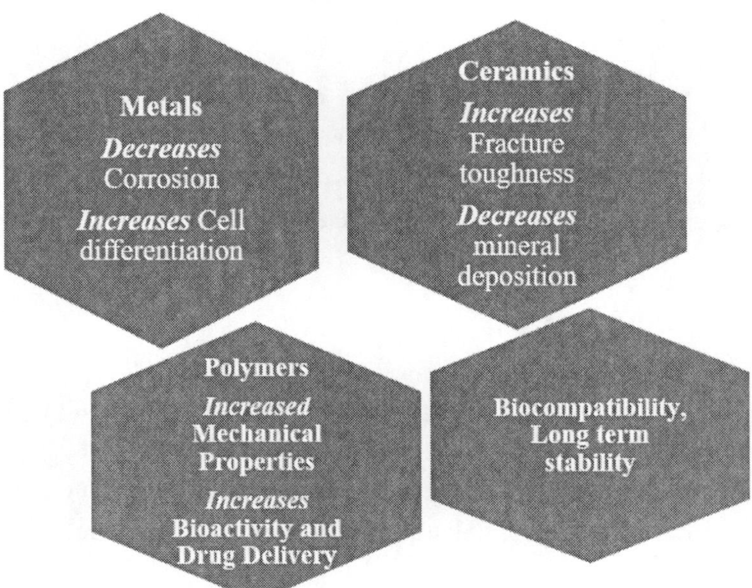

Figure 7. Possible improvements because of the incorporation of graphene in different biomaterials and identification of the key areas for making the concept of bio-composites a clinical reality.

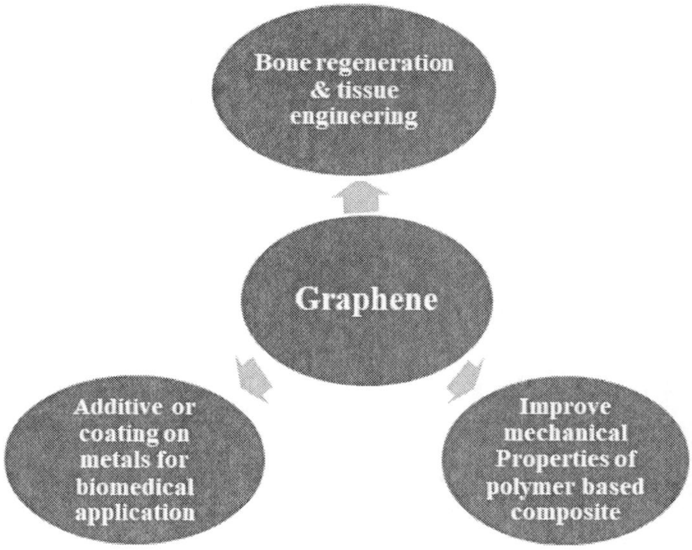

Figure 8. Applications of graphene in dentistry.

3.1.2. Graphene

Graphene is mostly found in two popular forms, namely graphene oxide (GO) and reduced graphene oxide (rGO). The residence of graphene-related materials and the ease with which they can be functionalized and combined with biomolecules and substances, opens up numerous possibilities to design bio- composites with tailored properties (Figure 7) (Xie 2017, 765).

Graphene is widely used in bone regeneration and tissue engineering (Figure 8). It is widely applied on to the implant surface and other metals for biomedical application. It's widely used to enhance the mechanical properties of tooth colour restorative material like composites.

3.1.3. Hydroxy Apatite

One of the major inorganic based components of tooth is hydroxyapatite. Hydroxyapatite ($Ca_{10}(PO_4)_6(OH)_2$, HAp), which is a form of calcium phosphate, and is one of the most biocompatible materials, but the low mechanical characteristics have limited its application for load-bearing materials. Chemical bonding with the host tissue offers HAp a greater advantage in clinical applications compared to most other bone substitutes such as allografts or metallic implants. The main advantages of synthetic HAp are its biocompatibility, slow in-situ biodegradability, and good osteoconductive and osteoinductive capabilities. The various techniques utilised for the synthesis of HAp are;

- Powder processing
- Co precipitation
- Hydrothermal reaction
- Micro-emulsion
- Mechanochemical synthesis.

There is a significant need to use clean, non-toxic and environmentally friendly techniques, HAp powders have been extracted using bio-products such as cuttlefish shells, corals, naturally occurring gypsum, naturally occurring calcite and bovine bone. On analysing chemically, these products, which were referred to as bio-wastes, have been found to be excellent sources of calcium carbonate and calcium oxide. Daily, about a million-metric tonne of egg shells are disposed as bio-waste around the world. The shells of eggs are almost 11 % of the total weight of an egg, and are mostly composed of calcium carbonate and calcium phosphate, in addition to traces of organic materials. Eggshells are inexpensive, available in plenty and are otherwise thrown away and hence can be used as biocompatible materials on the human body during implantation, but they are not osteo-conductive (Zhou 2011, 2769).

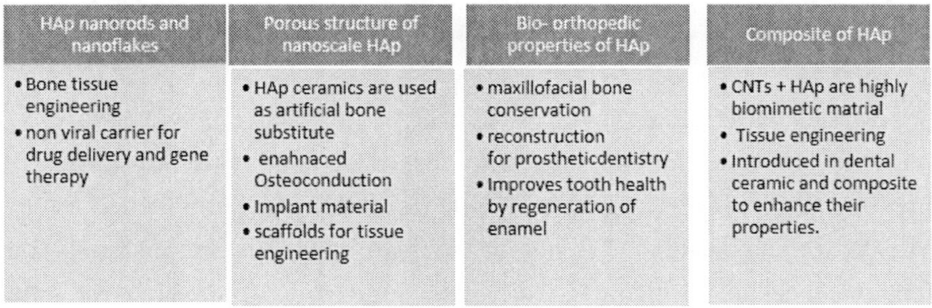

Figure 9. Application of HAp.

Hydroxyapatite nanorods and nano flakes are major components in non-viral drug delivery and gene therapy modalities (Figure 9). Since hydroxyapatite is naturally occurring in dentition and surrounding structures, HAp nanoparticles are, therefore, extensively used in regeneration of tooth enamel and bone.

3.1.4. Zirconia

Zirconia is a poly-crystalline, biocompatible, ceramic material, which has low reactivity with oral tissues and fluids, good resistance to wear and tear, and has excellent optical properties. It has been claimed by the manufacturers that the dioxide content in the ZLS glass-ceramics is about ten times higher as compared to other glass-ceramics. Hence, Zirconia is used for inlays, onlays, full-contour posterior and anterior crowns, and also in implant-supported prostheses (Figure 10) (Riquieri 2018, 1483). Zirconia monolithic crowns and prosthesis are used to replace any missing tooth. Their inert nature and high strength makes them ideal material to replace two or more teeth. There aesthetic appeal makes them highly acceptable material by the patient and the dentist.

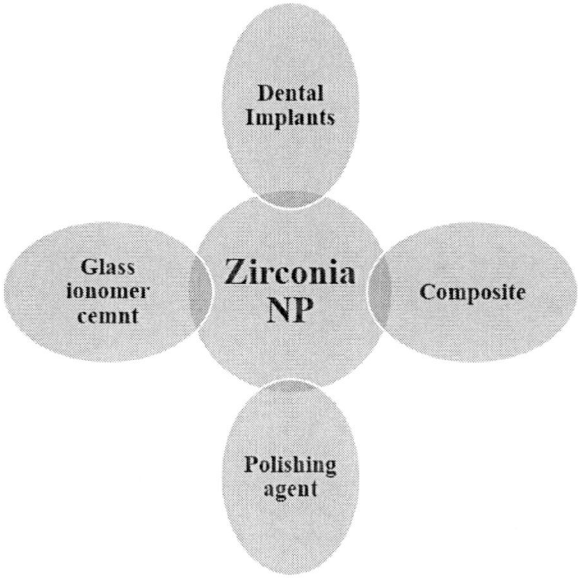

Figure 10. Applications of Zirconia in dentistry.

3.1.5. Silica

Silica NPs are extensively utilized in nanotechnology-based systems, as they are cost-effective and easy to fabricate. The specific surface properties, porosity and ability to customize the materials for easy fabrication, essentially make silica NPs good tools for detection of biomolecule and their separation, thereby giving solid media in drug delivery systems and also acting as protectors for contrast agents. Additionally, due to the biocompatibility and safety, they are employed as additives in various pharmaceuticals. SiNPs have wide applications in the detection of genes and gene purification, specifically because of their property to interact with nucleic acids. Using SiNPs in genetics has multiple advantages, like the usage of organic solvents, rapid processing and low costs. These days, the detection and extraction of DNA is being done for many diagnostic and therapeutic purposes. In dentistry, silica is commonly employed as fillers in different dental restorative materials. The uses of Si NPs have been illustrated in the following (Figure 11) (Bitar 2012, 1147).

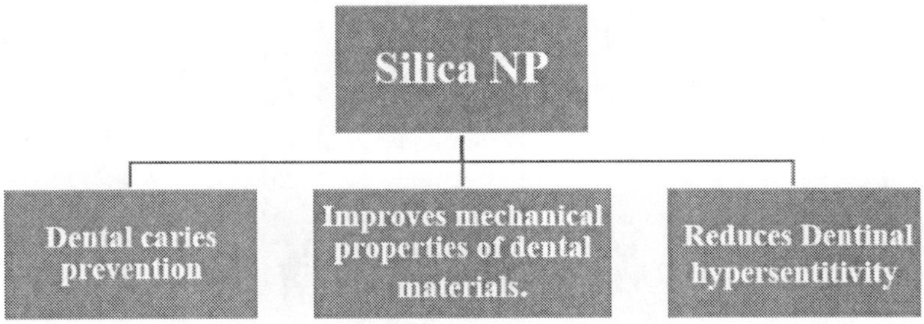

Figure 11. Applications Silica nanoparticles in dentistry.

3.1.6. Titania

Titanium has been widely accepted as a bone reparative material which has profound applications in orthopaedics, surgery and also in dentistry. Since titanium has a high resistance to fracture, has good ductile strength and high weight to strength ratio, it is one of the most sought-after materials. However, it does not possess bio-active properties such as enhancing cell adhesion and cell growth support. But when coated with apatite, titanium becomes bio-active and the bonding with bone tremendously increases leading to good osseointegration (Salata 2004, 3). When apatite is used as nanotubes on the surface of titanium, conjugated with zinc oxide nanoparticles (ZnO NPs), it becomes an excellent material suitable for the manufacture of dental implants.

ZnO NPs with size 20 to 50 nm have been bonded on the walls the TiO_2 nanotubes, acquiring anti-bacterial activity against streptococcus mutans and porphyromonas gingivalis through a steady and relaxed release of zinc ions. For tooth whitening, hydrogen peroxide has been conventionally used and recently, TiO_2 NPs are being used to increase the bleaching effects of hydrogen peroxide. Typical configurations utilised in nano-bio materials applied to medical or biological problems.

3.1.7. Silver Nanoparticles

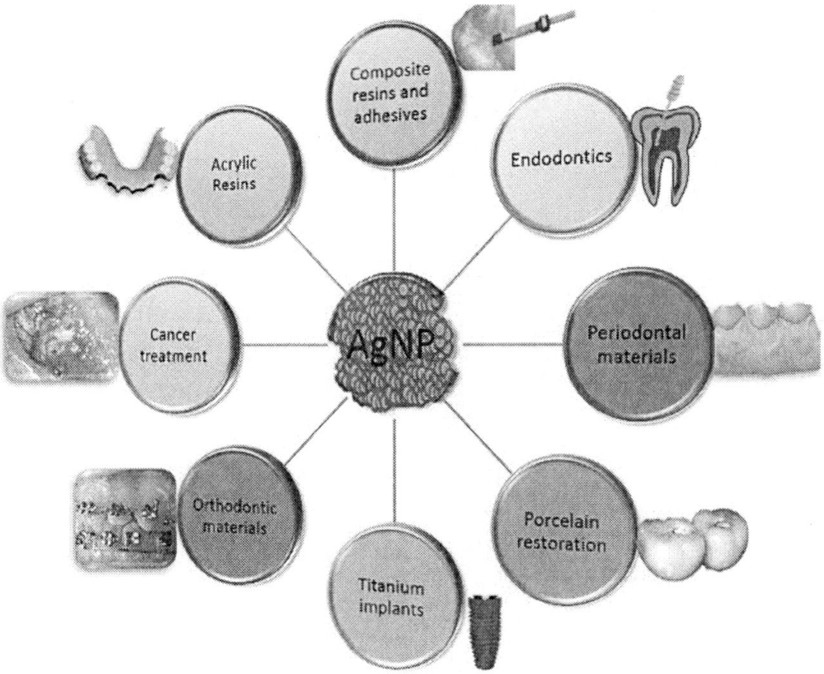

Figure 12. Silver NPs in dentistry.

The widespread use of silver in dentistry has been known for centuries with a world-wide acceptance of the precious metal since the 19th century.

Silver has formed a major component since then in the dental restorative material, i.e., the silver amalgam restoration. After 1930, the usage of silver amalgam restorations declined, on being substituted by tooth-coloured, aesthetically more acceptable, polymer-based resins. Silver nanoparticles (AgNPs) have been combined into different biomaterials for decreasing or preventing the formation of biofilm on the teeth surfaces (Figure 12). Because of the high surface to volume ratio with a tiny dimension of the particles, they acquired the most excellent antibacterial properties without diminishing any mechanical properties. Due to this special property of these Ag NPs, the nano-filled materials are the gold standard for use as fillers in different biomaterials, as the efficacy and function increases substantially (Bapat 2018, 881).

3.2. Organic Nanoparticles

3.2.1. Chitosan

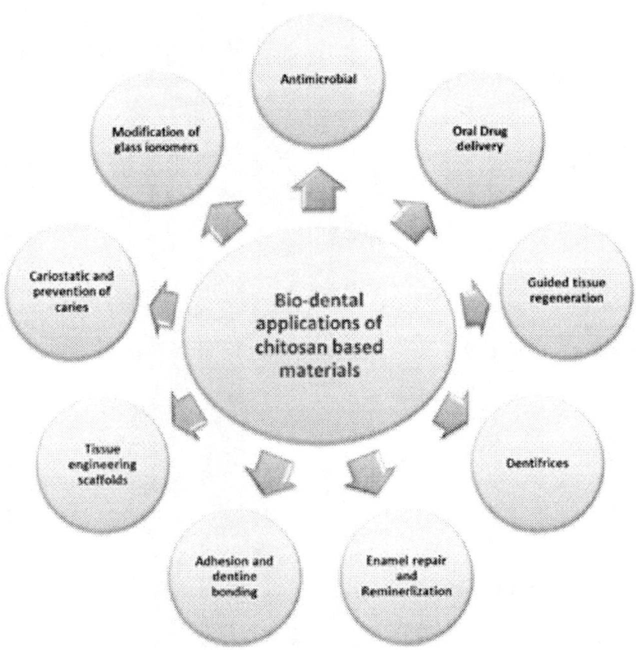
Antimicrobial
Oral Drug delivery
Guided tissue regeneration
Dentifrices
Enamel repair and Reminerlization
Adhesion and dentine bonding
Tissue engineering scaffolds
Cariostatic and prevention of caries
Modification of glass ionomers
Bio-dental applications of chitosan based materials

Figure 13. Current and potential application of chitosan in dentistry.

Chitosan (CHS) is a naturally occurring dynamic biomaterial which has recently been used for a variety of applications in dentistry (Figure 13). CHS has multiple advantages as a biomaterial due to its properties like biocompatibility, hydrophilicity, biodegradability, and a broad spectrum of antimicrobial activity (encompassing gram-negative and gram-positive bacteria and also fungi). Moreover, the molecular structure of CHS possesses reactive functional groups which give multiple reactive sites and chances for the formation of electro-chemical relationships at the cell and molecular level. These special properties of CHS have garnered the attention of material scientists around the world for exploring its increasing bio-dental uses (Husain 2017, 602).

4. Nanotechnology in Restorative Dentistry

Table 4. Nanotechnology-based strategies for combating oral biofilms and dental caries

Restorative material	Nanoparticles added	Function
Composite resin; Dental primer; Dental adhesive	Silver nanoparticles	Antimicrobial
Composite resin	Zinc oxide nanoparticles	Antimicrobial
Composite resin; Glass ionomer cement	Quaternary ammonium polyethylenimine (QAS-PEI)	Antimicrobial
Composite resin; Dental adhesive; Glass ionomer cement	Calcium phosphate ($CaPO_4$) nanoparticles	Remineralizing
Composite resin	Calcium fluoride (CaF_2) nanoparticles	Remineralizing
Resin modified GIC (RMGIC)	Nanohydroxyapatite (nano-HA) or nano fluoro hydroxyapatite (nano-FHA)	Remineralizing

Metals, polymers, ceramics and composites are the four major kinds of dental materials used in dentistry for restorations (Table 2). The above categories of dental materials have now incorporated nanotechnology for practical applications in restorative dentistry. Because of their unique properties, these nanomaterials are a source of experimentation for achieving better biomaterials to be used in dentistry (Khursh 2015, 717).

4.1. Nanocomposite

Presently, nanotechnology has its dominant effect on restorative dentistry by means of offering refinements to already clinically established resin-based composite structures. Nanohybrid and nanofilled resin-based composites are generally the two kinds of restorative substances noted as "nanocomposite," commonly in a context of particle size. These are characterized by using filler-particle having sizes of ≤ 100 nm, and these substances can provide aesthetic and electricity advantages over conventional microfilled and hybrid resin-based composite systems, broadly speaking in terms of smoothness, polishability and precision of shade characterization, plus flexural electricity and microhardness just like those of the higher-acting posterior resin-based composites (Figure 14). Due to the metal free tagging, composite resins can mimic most of the natural tooth shades, more so in the highly aesthetically demanding anterior regions, thereby fulfilling the patient's persistent demands for a "teeth-like" restoration (Sachdeva 2015, 52). Composites are composed of three distinct phases, each with its own role in dictating material properties: the polymerizable resin, filler, and the filler-resin interface. Composites comprise of three unique phases, each with possessing its role in dictating the properties of the materials: the polymerizable resin, filler, and the filler-resin interface. The radical technique of nanotechnology has enabled incorporation of nanofiller particles in the healthy resin matrix of dental composites at a nano-scale, leading to a mammoth improvement in mechanical, aesthetic and optical properties, as compared to those of the traditional, microfilled and hybrid resins (Sachdeva 2015, 52).

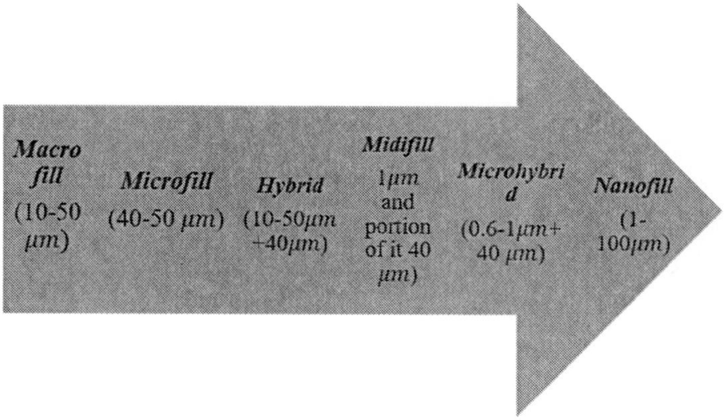

Figure 14. Chronological development of resin composite.

Advantages of nanocomposite over conventional/traditional composites are:

- Improved aesthetic
- Improved optical properties
- Precision of shade characterization
- Colour stability
- Provides excellent gloss and finish
- High polish retention post tooth brush abrasion
- Greater modulus of elasticity
- Higher flexural, tensile and impact strength.
- Reduced viscosity
- Increase hardness.

Nanocomposites are available in nanohybrid and nanofill as dental restorative material. There are numerous brands of nanocomposites which are now commercially available including, Filtek Supreme XTE Universal Restorative (3M ESPE), Premise (Kerr/Sybron, Orange, CA), IPS Empress Direct & Tetric N-Ceram (both Ivoclar Vivadent) etc. (Sachdeva S 2015). Recently, a systematic review which is authored by Alzraikat et al., studied the properties of nanocomposite resin and their efficacy in a clinical settings. They came to a conclusion that the filler loading and the presence of nanofiller could change the viscoelastic conduct of the composite substances as well as macrophage cell adhesion, despite the fact that editions in the methacrylate conversion produced probably the most massive differences.

4.2. Nano Glass Ionomers

Glass ionomers were introduced by Wilson and Kent in the 1070s, as a dental restorative material. Glass ionomers are being used broadly because of their high-quality properties akin to chemical bonding to the tooth constitution, biocompatibility and fluoride release. On the other hand, there are a number of shortcomings for this group of substances, reminiscent of negative aesthetic, prolonged setting response, compromised mechanical properties and weaker bond. To improve these properties and to address the shortcomings, active ongoing research, such as the addition of cellulose fibers, hydroxyapatite and fluoroapatite and nanotechnologies, are going on.

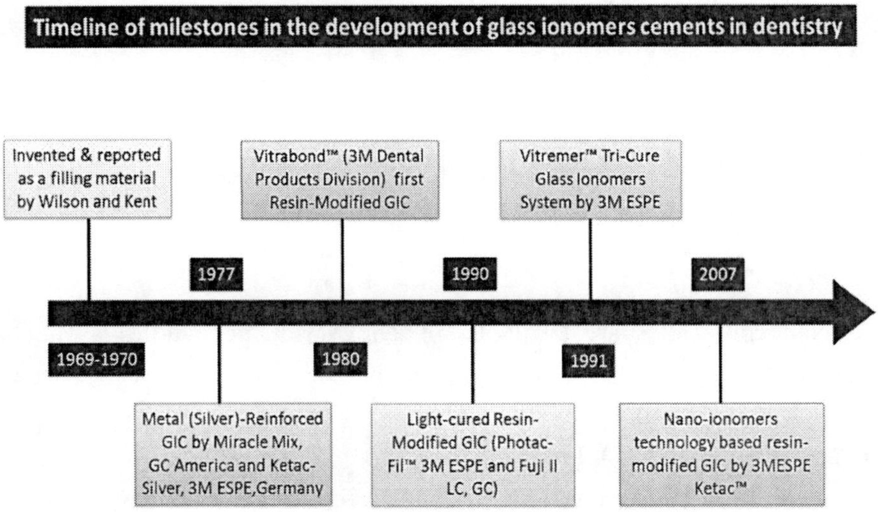

Figure 15. Development of glass ionomer restorative material.

Table 5. Composition of traditional GIC with Nanofill GIC

	Traditional GIC	Nanofill GIC
Composition	a) Powder: fluoro-aluminosilicate glass and aqueous solution containing polyalkenoic acids which are carboxylic acids b) Liquid: Polyacrylic acid, tartaric acid c) Other additives: Ba- and Sr-salts	1) Powder Modified Nano Glass Ionomer: Nanosized Glass particles 2) Nano – Apatite : nHAp or nano-fluoroapatite (nFAp) 3) Modification with Nano-Sized HAp/Zr, $CaF2$ and $TiO2$ Particles 4) Nano-Filled Resin-Modified Glass Ionomer Cements

Advantages of nanofill glass Ionomer over traditional composite:

- More desirable ease of handling and manipulation
- Cut back the treatment time, benefitting both the clinician as well as the patient
- Improving the mechanical properties adds to the serviceability and self-life of restorative substances as they are capable to withstand the masticatory and occlusal forces more effectively.
- Nano-apatite containing glass ionomers are expected to have advanced bonding to the tooth surface.
- Enhanced fluoride liberation, which aids in anti-cariogenic capability.

4.3. Nano-Adhesives

Creating and preserving a strong and long lasting adhesive joint between resin composite restorations and enamel and dentin teeth substrates by using today's adhesive programs is regarded a fundamental goal in restorative dentistry. The degradation of the bond with age is manifested clinically via caries recurrence, which is the principal intent of restoration alternative. Significant efforts have been made to enhance the sturdiness of the resin–dentin bond and strengthen the longevity of resin-based restorations. Amongst these methods, foremost is the development of the properties of the adhesive material with the aid of fortifying it with nanoparticles. Nanotechnology and nanoscience have prepared the ground by the processing of considerable varieties of nanofillers that pose further organic advantages, like competent antimicrobial and remineralizing capability (Dina Elkassas 2017, 1543). There are numerous therapeutic nanoparticles incorporated in dental adhesives depending on the site where desired effect is required.

Adhesives with antimicrobial properties contain silver. In some cases, when the pulp tissue gets damaged due to iatrogenic causes, the dental adhesives with hydroxyapatite, bioactive glass or amorphous calcium phosphate are used to form dentinal bridge. This dentinal bridge aids in healing of the pulp and restores the vitality of the tooth. Other uses are listed in Figure 16.

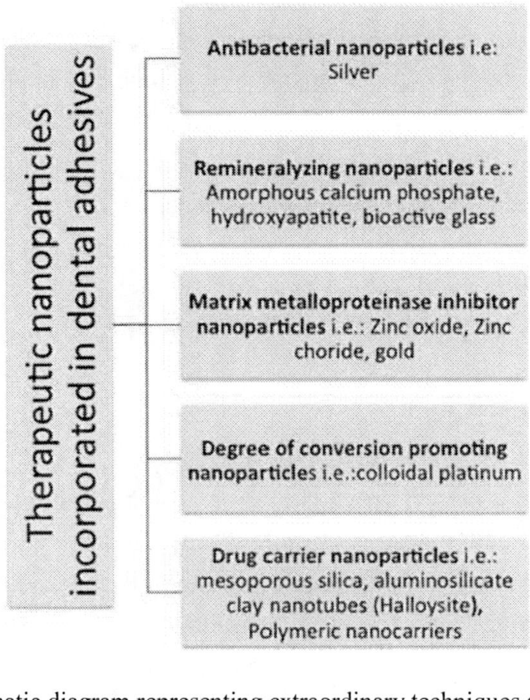

Figure 16. Schematic diagram representing extraordinary techniques adopted in the nanoparticles technology to increase adhesive joint durability.

4.4. Local Anaesthesia

Most of the patients undergoing restorative treatment have to go through pain during the procedure. To overcome this hurdle, and to ensure patient's comfort during the treatment, local anaesthetics (LA) are administered. This LA makes the operative area numb, which can last for approximately 1-3 hrs. The LA is deposited via needle and syringe technique at a place, where the nerve innervation supply to the tooth and surrounding tissue occur. This can lead to anxiety and patient might be unwilling to undergo the procedure. Nanotechnology aids in overcoming this fear and enables lengthy hours of working (Moradkhani 2018, 355).

Strategies are adopted to obtain controlled release of LA at the site of administration. Polymeric micro and nanoparticles had been used as administration techniques for more than a few local anaesthetic agents. These systems can deliver relatively significant quantities of drug in comparison to aqueous solutions and can unlock them over prolonged periods. Conventional regional anaesthetics can be included into such polymeric substances (e.g., with the aid of single emulsion) with ease, especially seeing that their free bases and the polymer matrix will also be dissolved in commonly available organic solvents. In some cases, systemic toxicity appears to be problematic, however local toxicity is a greater hassle with most, in particular with delivery of amino-amide and amino-ester local anaesthetics (Santamaria 2017, 22).

5. Nanotechnology Applications in Periodontics

Periodontics is a branch of science which deals with the health of surrounding structures of a tooth. The oral hygiene aids in promoting good oral health. Improper brushing technique is detrimental to both tooth and its supporting structures. Periodontal diseases can lead to:

- Bleeding gums
- Pockets

- Gingival recession
- Loose teeth due to decrease in the bone level
- Foul smell from mouth/Halitosis
- Increased spacing between tooth/pathological migration

5.1. Dentinal Hypersensitivity

Dentinal hypersensitivity is characterized by quick, sharp suffering coming up from exposed dentine in accordance with stimuli such as thermal, evaporative, tactile, osmotic or chemical and which can't be ascribed to another form of dental defect or pathology. Dentine can be exposed as a result of gingival recession. Carbonated hydroxyapatite nanocrystals synthesized with tailor-made biomimetic characteristics for composition, constitution, size and morphology, can chemically bind themselves on the surfaces of enamel tissues, fill the scratches, produce a bound biomimetic apatitic coating and can defend the enamel surface constitution. These nanoparticles are incorporated in specially formulated tooth-pastes. These occlude the dentinal tubules or form a protective barrier on sensitive tooth, which enables tooth to be non-responsive to thermal stimuli. Some strategies to manage the dentinal hypersensitivity is presented in the following Figure (Figure 17).

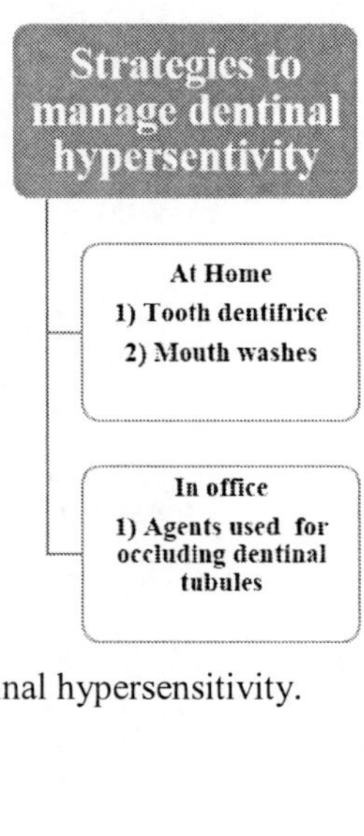

Figure 17. Treatment for dentinal hypersensitivity.

5.2. Tooth Dentifrice and Mouth Wash

Dentifrices are the most commonly used dental desensitizing agents because of their low price, ease of use, and house application. When nano-hydroxyapatite is used in toothpaste, it forms a protecting film on the tooth enamel, and even helps restore the outside broken areas. The nano-hydroxyapatite aid in remineralization and thereby occludes dentinal tubules. The clinical trial comparing tooth paste containing NovaMin and nano-HAP showed significant reductions in dentine hypersensitivity at the end of 4 weeks (Gopinath 2015, 118).

5.3. Current Applications of Nanoparticles in Periodontics

Nanotechnology offers a novel local drug delivery method, adequate for the cure of periodontal diseases (Figure 18). The microspheres can also be directly positioned in the pockets or at the place of gingival inflammation and might act locally to control the progression of ailment. Nanotechnology and its usage in periodontics have greatly improved the diagnosis, medication, prognosis and prevention of the periodontal diseases. It utilizes nanomaterials, nanobiotechnology and nanorobots for the treatment and preservation of periodontal wellbeing. They also enable local drug delivery to the target tissues, cells, or subcellular compartments in periodontal pockets, to both biofilm pathogens and host cells, as well as control the discharge of included drugs, which are almost always antibiotic or anti-inflammatory ones. Particular examples of the nano-carriers or nanomaterials such as liposomes, lipid and polymeric nanoparticles, nanocrystals, dendrimers, and nanofibers are being constantly and actively monitored for their effectiveness in healing periodontal disorders. Nanofibers are of distinctive interest as nano-delivery methods and scaffolds for the regeneration of periodontal tissue (Khetawat 2015, 181).

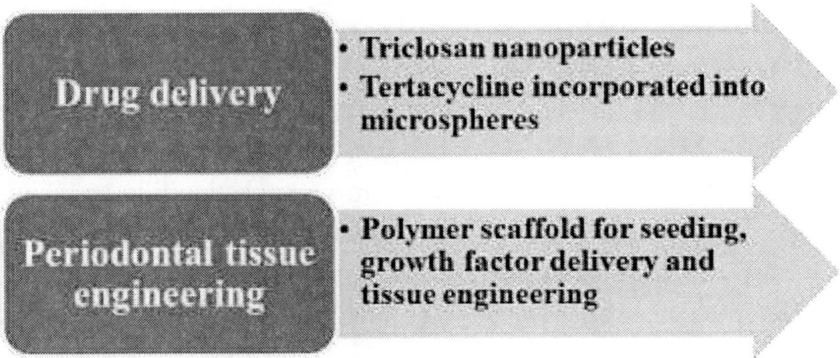

Figure 18. Application of nanotechnology in branch of periodontics.

6. Nanotechnology in Endodontics

Endodontics is the branch of dentistry which deals with the diseases of pulp. It maintains the tooth in its natural position and arch. A primary test in root canal cure is the inability of the present cleaning and shaping procedures to do away with bacterial biofilms surviving inside the anatomic complexities, and un-instrumented parts of the root canal system. On account of the shortcomings of current anti-biofilm methods in root canal treatment, newer disinfection methods are being developed and experimented. These disinfecting materials can be in the form of irrigants, which are used to clean the root canal. They can also be incorporated in obturating materials or sealer to provide antibacterial effect and fluid tight seal (Nazila Akbarianrad 2018, 121).

6.1. Nano Based Irrigating Solution

Irrigating solutions are routinely used in root canal therapy to clean canals of organic and inorganic debris. It reduces the microbiological burden within the root canals.

Table 6. Difference between conventional and nanoparticle irrigating solutions

Conventional irrigating solution (like NaOCl)	**Irrigating solution with Nanoparticles**
It does not penetrate to small confines of root canal anatomy	Penetrates to smallest intricate parts of root canal
Poor smear layer removal capacity	Active against both inorganic and organic components of root canal
Not much effective against E. faecalis	Effective against E. faecalis.

6.2. Nanoparticles in Endodontic Sealers

The most important purpose of root canal therapy is to create a 3-dimensional seal. It is performed by using sealers and obturating substances. Thus, root canal sealers with just the right amount of sealing capability and longer antimicrobial activity are desirable. Additionally, antibacterial endodontic sealers should be lethal against contaminating bacteria without harming enamel-supporting tissues. Incorporation of quaternary ammonium poly (ethylenimine) (QPEI) nanoparticles into non-cytotoxic endodontic sealers akin to silicon-based sealers could go a long way in enhancing the antibacterial properties without compromising the materials' biocompatibility. Incorporation of zinc and silver nanoparticles improved the flowability of the endodontic sealer substances. The small size of nanoparticles ensures that they can penetrate dentinal tubules to seal all areas effortlessly; the development of a sealer, based on nanotechnology, is the most important step to gain a better sealer in endodontics. These substances are biocompatible, antimicrobial, and possess biomineralization.

6.3. Nanotechnology Software in Regeneration of Pulp Tissue

Nanotechnologies optimize the distribution of active molecules and the extracellular mimetic structure of scaffolds. For this reason, they appear essential to control/inhibit illness and infection and orchestrate pulp cell colonization and differentiation. In the future, nanotechnologies would be in a position to build temporally and spatially managed drug supply methods of several primary bioactive molecules. These multi-functionalized nanomaterials would effectively address the challenges of problematic dental pulp regeneration (Keller 2015, 7461).

7. Nanotechnology in Orthodontics

Orthodontics is a branch which deals with the correction of the occlusion of the patient. It ensures correct alignment of teeth within the jaw. By adding nano-particles to the materials employed in orthodontics, their mechanical properties such as shear bonding strength can be enhanced. Additionally, the nanoparticles are applied in orthodontics as shown in the following Figure (Figure 19).

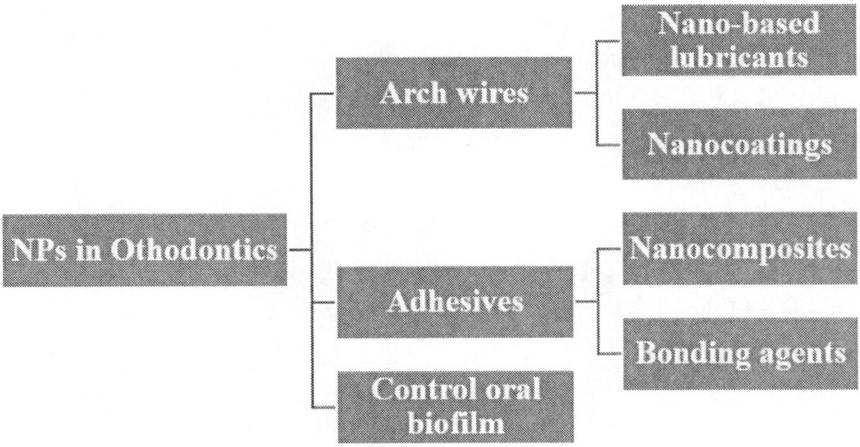

Figure 19. Application of nano-particles in orthodontics.

7.1. Arch Wires

Table 7. Types of arch wire

Type of arch wire	Nano coating and nanolubricant
Nickel Titanium	Tungsten disulfide (WS_2)
Stainless steel	Composite Coating of Co and Fullerene like WS_2 Carbon Nitride (CNx) ZnO Molybdenum Disulphide NPs Nanostructured DLC coating
Hollow wires	NiTi/$NiTiO_2$ Composite NPs

Arch wires are coated with nano-particles to reduce friction. Friction interferes with the forces applied onto the tooth, thereby hindering the proper alignment of teeth (Batra 2016).

7.2. Orthodontic Brackets

The orthodontic brackets are placed on the tooth using adhesives and flowable composite resin. The problem with orthodontic bracket placement on tooth is that after a span of 1- 2 years, it has been observed that an isolated white spot appears, which were previously occupied by these brackets. These orthodontic brackets can be;

1. Metallic
2. Non metallic

These white spot lesions are hypo-mineralised zone which are prone to caries. Strategies have been adopted to make adhesives and composites which are antimicrobial as well as remineralizing. The nanotechnology-based applications in orthodontic materials have been widely reported in the literature over the past few years. However, the number of studies which have specifically addressed orthodontics and nanotechnology are limited. In the near future, there would be a significant increase in the amount and quality of translational research that will reveal the newer generation of nanomaterials for orthodontic treatment.

Table 8. Nanoparticles' application in orthodontics

Antimicrobial NPs	Enamel remineralizing NPs
Nitrogen doped titanium oxide brackets	Calcium nanophosphate
Fluoroapatite, Fluorohydroxyapatite, Hydroxyapatite.	Nano Hydroxy apatite
Chitosan	Fluoride
Copper	
Fluoride releasing NPs	
Silver	
Quaternary ammonia dimethyl amino do decyl methaacrylate	

8. Nanoparticles Applications in Oral Maxillofacial Surgery

Oral and maxillofacial surgery involves detection, surgical intervention and restoring realistic and aesthetic facets of difficult and delicate tissues in the head and neck region. Regenerative nanotechnology is at the forefront of scientific study, and translational remedy is a mission to each scientists and clinicians. There has been an exponential upward thrust within the quantity of study carried out in this field, for both surgical and medicinal uses. In the field of oral and maxillofacial surgery, nano-technology has influenced the development of tissue engineering, imaging, delivery of medicinal drugs, and has improved implants.

8.1. Nanoscaffolds for Tissue Engineering

Harvesting bone from autologous or allograft donor sites is a highly-priced and invasive approach, which is related to extra surgical procedures.

Tissue engineering systems contain the mixture of cells, biomaterial scaffolds and specialized culture conditions incorporating biochemical and physical stimuli to motivate in-vitro bone formation. The perfect method for regenerative bone treatment plans is to use a "smart" biomaterial scaffold that may modulate the procedure of remedy while providing mechanical support.

The various nanomaterials, used in the bone reconstruction, are: derivatives of polyhydroxyacids, such as polylactide (PLA), polyglycolide (PGA), poly(ε-caprolactone) (PCL), and their copolymers poly (lactide-co-glycolide) (PLGA), poly(lactide-co-caprolactone) (PLC), poly(glycolide-cocaprolactone) (PGC), and poly(L-lactic acid) (PLLA) (He 2009, 63).

Regenerative nanotechnology-based uses in oral and maxillofacial surgery are growing fast and there are a number of recent developments too. The field of biomaterials used for bone regeneration is already well acclaimed, but the use of nanoscience and nanotechnology, especially for oral and maxillofacial surgery is still evolving (Figure 20). There are two broad areas of research using nanotechnology based systems: the use of multi-functional theranostic (diagnostic as well as therapeutic) nanoparticles for oral malignancies, and utility of nano-inspired biomaterials for enhancing regeneration of bone, particularly for oral and maxillofacial surgery.

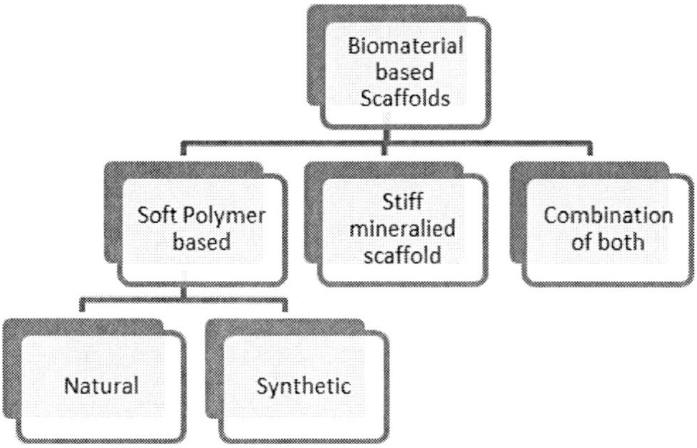

Figure 20. Two distinct biomaterial-based approaches support stem cell-based bone regeneration.

Table 9. Commercially available scaffolds for human use

Nanomaterial	Application
Nano-structured magnesium – hydroxyapatite and Human demineralised bone matric	Repair of bony defects and generation of new bone.
Polycaprolactone (PCL)-based	Reconstruction of craniofacial region
NanoBone®	Used in sinus lift

9. Application in Prosthodontics

Prosthodontics is the branch of dentistry that mainly deals with the replacement of lost tooth and tissue structures of oral cavity with dentures and crowns. It also includes fabrication of custom-made prostheses for temporomandibular joint disabilities, and maxilla-facial tissue deformities. Most of the dental materials used today are formulated through nano-crystallization to enhance their original activity and to play a pivotal role in different oral applications. Research in dental materials based on nanotechnology encompasses two main pathways: preparation of new inorganic nanoparticles and alteration of the surface of the existing bio-materials with the use of inorganic nanofillers.

9.1. Nanoresin

The impregnation of nanofillers has significantly changed some properties like surface hardness, modulus of elasticity, filler loading and polymerization shrinkage, in the case of composite resins. Nano-filled denture bases have greater inter-facial shear bond strength in between the resin matrix and nanofillers, as compared to the resin matrix used in conventional composites. The super-molecular bonding encloses or coats the nano-materials, thereby making a thicker interface and increases the bonding between the different resin molecules leading to a higher molecular weight polymerized resin. Poly (methyl methacrylate) (PMMA) is one of the most widely used biomaterial for manufacturing denture prosthesis in dentistry. It has been observed that Candida albicans is almost invariably present in about 60% of the removable denture wearers. PMMA, synthesised with nano-pigments is not only biocompatible but it has various advantages considering its physical properties, which impedes the colonization of Candida albicans onto the denture (Gad 2019). Even silver nanoparticles have been impregnated onto the PMMA denture resin, for acquiring a possible anti-microbial effect onto the denture so that common oral infections are prevented in removable denture wearers and a healthy oral environment is maintained (Monteiro 2012, 7).

9.2. Nanoceramics

The most crucial physical properties of denture teeth used inside the restoration of the edentulous person is wear resistance. Immoderate wear of acrylic resin teeth has been a challenge to each of the affected person and the dentist because of unfavourable related sequelae. Nanoceramic refers to the ceramic material with nanoscale dimensions within the microstructures segment. Persson et al. reported that as compared to the conventional ceramics, nanoceramics have unique properties; first of all, nanoceramics have splendid plasticity. Ceramic is a kind of brittle substance; however, nanoceramic possesses excellent durability and ductility. The association of atoms in nanoceramics interface is quite unclear; the atoms are very clean to migrate underneath the situations of force deformation. Secondly, in comparison to the conventional ceramics, nanoceramic has far more advanced mechanical properties, inclusive of substantial sturdiness and hardness. The hardness and sturdiness of many nanoceramics are four to five times better than the traditional substances.

The only drawback is that it causes excessive wearing of the opposing natural teeth and the clicking sound generated off the ceramic teeth (Persson 2012, 4105). To overcome this, nano composite teeth are introduced, which are harder and more wear resistant than the acrylic teeth. They are also compatible with the opposing natural tooth.

9.3. Nanotechnology in Impression Materials

Nanoparticles are integrated in vinylpolysiloxanes, an addition reaction, silicone elastomer impression material go through to produce a material which has better flow, improved hydrophilic properties and has lesser voids at the margin, easier pouring of models with excellent reproduction of details.

10. NANOTECHNOLOGY IN IMPLANTS

Dental implants are now the most common prosthesis used in dentistry for the replacement of missing teeth. However, the field of implantology is not without challenges, especially considering the osseointegration between the implant and the alveolar bone and the preservation of the integrity of the epithelial junction of the gingiva. The ongoing research in dentistry involves structural modifications in the dental implant surfaces so that better osseointegration is achieved (Figure 21).

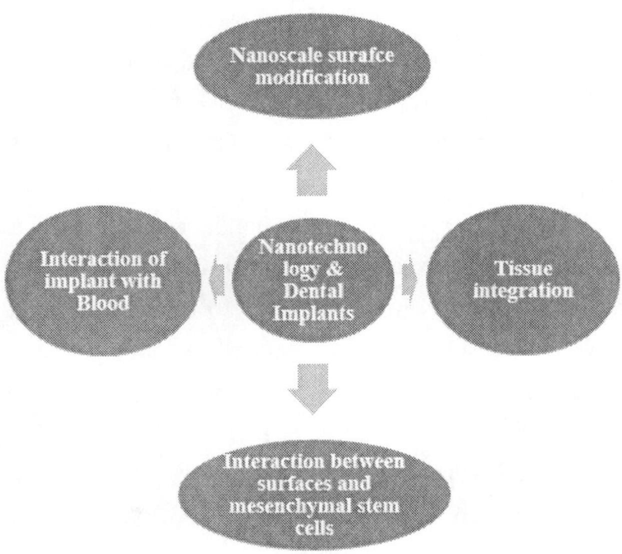

Figure 21. The different steps of the interactions between biological fluids, cells, tissues, and surfaces of implants.

The principal objective is to create a metallic implant surface with biological properties for the adsorption of proteins, enabling adherence, cell differentiation as well as tissue integration. Nanotechnology may help in the production of controlled topography and chemistry, which will help in understanding biological interactions and development of unique implant surfaces with favourable tissue-integrative properties (Tomsia 2013, 28).

Table 10. Nanosurface coating on implants

Surface Treatment	Nano technology technique	Properties
Anodic oxidation	Nanotubes and nano hydroxyapatite coating	Improves bioactivity
Acid treatment	Titanium is etched with HCL and forms nanopits	Antimicrobial efficacy can be enhanced by incorporating Fluorine in these pits. Contributed to bone regeneration
Alkali Treatment	Implant is immersed in sodium and potassium hydroxide followed by heat treatment. This results in growth of nanostructured and bioactive sodium titanate layer.	Provides favourable condition for bone marrow cell differentiation
Combination of Anodization and chemical etching	Anodised nano tubular Ti is coated with NaOH treated PLGA.	Stimulates cell activity
Hydrogen peroxide treatment	Dissolution and oxidation of implant	Makes it more receptive for deposition of nano HP NPs
Sol- gel method	deposition of discrete 20-40 nm nanoparticles on a dual acid-etched implant surface	High bond strength between implant surface and nanoscale coating is due to high electron density at atomic level.

Advantages of creating nano-roughness on titanium implants

- Increment in surface area of the implants adjacent to the bone.
- Better attachment of cells to the surface of the implants.
- Enhancement of bone present at the implant site.
- 4. The bio-mechanical compatibility between the dental implants and alveolar bone is better.

Many in vivo and in vitro studies have shown that different unique dental implant surfaces could be fabricated mostly consisting of different modifications in commercially available implants. Nano surface modification methods are likely to enhance surface properties of titanium dental implants, which can magnify the peri-implant osteogenesis.

Table 11. The different techniques utilized for creation of bioactive nano-surface on biocompatible metal surfaces

Physical techniques	Nanoparticle used	Properties
Plasma spraying	Au, Ag, Ti, Calcium Phosphate (HA)	Enhanced bone implant contact
Sputtering	Hydroxyapatite and Calcum phosphate	greater adhesion between the coating and substrate along with greater control on properties of coating.
Ion implantation	Hydroxyapatite layer	Adhesion between implanted surface and substrate is excellent. This method of application is easily reproducible and controllable.
Thermal oxidation	Changes crystalline structure of nanometric oxide layer	Makes metal surface more biocompatible.

11. Toxicity Associated with Nanoparticles

The ability of a material to be used in conjunction with biological tissues or within the tissues without the production of any adverse effects locally or systemically is referred to as biocompatibility. While the advantages of the nanoparticles used for various purposes have been stressed upon, they are not without potential adverse effects. They may react differently when exposed to different environments. Because of their size, they can easily penetrate the cell membrane and bring about changes at the cellular level. An important criterion is the dosage for identification of hazards and assessment of risks for the usage of nanotechnology in dentistry. Hence, an in-depth understanding of the nanoparticle pathways and entry portals of the human body is essential for the facilitation of future research and formation of policy by regulatory bodies ought to take into consideration the toxic potential of the nanomaterials.

Table 12. Examples of metal nanoparticles and their associated toxic effects on cell

Nanoparticles	Associated effects
Ag NPs	Enhancement in reactive oxygen species (ROS) production, oxidative stress, damage to mitochondria and DNA and cytotoxicity in BRL 3A rat liver cells as well as human liver cells,
Titanium Oxide (TiO_2)	Increase in the formation of ROS in various mammalian cells

Conclusion

A significant step in nanotoxicology is the characterization of the nanomaterials under consideration, and this can be very troublesome than in the case in classical toxicology due to more number of variables in the parameter space. These include: size of the particle, roughness, shape, charge, composition and surface coating. The latter can deviate, based on the matrix into which it is incorporated. Deduction of the dose of the nanoparticle is complex, which needs many direct and/or indirect technologies for determining as to how many particles are entering defined targets. Like in other emerging fields, here too a regulatory framework needs to be developed based on the objective scientific research that can help in limiting the exposure of humans to potentially hazardous engineered nanomaterials, that too by keeping the environment safe. However, the therapeutic use of nanomaterials in dentistry and medicine requires the usage of a different framework to bring a balance between the treatment benefits and the supposed harmful effects (Andreas Elsaesser 2012, 129).

REFERENCES

Abramovitz, I., Beyth, N., Weinberg, G., Borenstein, A., Polak, D., Kesler-Shvero, D., & Houri-Haddad, Y. (2012). In vitro biocompatibility of endodontic sealers incorporating antibacterial nanoparticles. *Journal of Nanomaterials, 2012*, 12. doi: 10.1155/2012/858073.

Akasaka, T., Nakata, K., Uo, M., & Watari, F. 2009. "Modification of the dentin surface by using carbon nanotubes." *Bio-medical materials and engineering*, 19: 179-185. doi: 10.3233/BME-2009-0578.

Akbarianrad, N., Mohammadian, F., Alhuyi Nazari, M., & Rahbani Nobar, B. 2018. "Applications of nanotechnology in endodontic: A Review." *Nanomedicine Journal*, 5: 121-126. doi: 10.22038/NMJ.2018.005.00 01.

AlKahtani, R. N. 2018. "The implications and applications of nanotechnology in dentistry: A review." *The Saudi dental journal*, 30: 107-116. doi: 10.1016/j.sdentj.2018.01.002.

Bapat, R. A., Chaubal, T. V., Joshi, C. P., Bapat, P. R., Choudhury, H., Pandey, M., Gorain, B., & Kesharwani, P. 2018. "An overview of application of silver nanoparticles for biomaterials in dentistry." *Materials Science and Engineering: C*, 91, 881-898. doi: 10.1016/j.m sec.2018.05.069.

Batra, P., Mushtaq, A., Mazumder, M., Rizvi, M. S., and Miglani, R. 2016. "Nanoparticles and their Applications in Orthodontics." *Adv Dent & Oral Health* 2.

Bitar, A., Ahmad, N. M., Fessi, H., & Elaissari, A. 2012. "Silica-based nanoparticles for biomedical applications." *Drug discovery today*, 17: 1147-1154. doi: 10.1016/j.drudis.2012.06.014.

Chaloupka, K., Malam, Y., & Seifalian, A. M. 2010. "Nanosilver as a new generation of nanoproduct in biomedical applications." *Trends in biotechnology*, 28: 580-588. doi: 10.1016/j.tibtech.2010.07.006.

Elkassas, D., & Arafa, A. 2017. "The innovative applications of therapeutic nanostructures in dentistry." *Nanomedicine: Nanotechnology, Biology and Medicine*, 13: 1543-1562. doi: 10.1016 /j.nano.2017.01.018.

ElKateb, W. M., Massoud, A. G., Mokhless, N. A., Shalaby, T. I. "Measurement of Tubular Penetration Depth of Three Types of Nanoparticles Mixed With Endodontic Sealer Using Scanning Electron Microscope An *In Vitro* Study." *Journal of American Science*, 11.

Elsaesser, A., & Howard, C. V. 2012. "Toxicology of nanoparticles." *Advanced drug delivery reviews*, 64: 129-137. doi: 10.1016/j.addr.2011.09.001.

Fernandez-Yague, M. A., Abbah, S. A., McNamara, L., Zeugolis, D. I., Pandit, A., & Biggs, M. J. 2015. "Biomimetic approaches in bone tissue engineering: Integrating biological and physicomechanical strategies." *Advanced drug delivery reviews*, 84: 1-29. doi: 10.1016/j.addr.2014.09.005.

Gad, M. M., & Abualsaud, R. 2019. "Behavior of PMMA Denture Base Materials Containing Titanium Dioxide Nanoparticles: A Literature Review." *International journal of biomaterials*, 2019. doi: 10.1155/2019/6190610.

Gopinath, N. M., John, J., Nagappan, N., Prabhu, S., & Kumar, E. S. 2015. "Evaluation of dentifrice containing nano-hydroxyapatite for dentinal hypersensitivity: a randomized controlled trial." *Journal of international oral health: JIOH*, 7: 118. URL: https://www.ncbi.nlm.nih.gov/pmc/articles/PMC4588776/.

Guggenberger, R., May, R., & Stefan, K. P. 1998. "New trends in glass-ionomer chemistry." *Biomaterials*, 19: 479-483. doi: 10.1016/S0142-9612(97)00127-0.

Hamouda, I. M. 2012. "Current perspectives of nanoparticles in medical and dental biomaterials." *Journal of biomedical research*, 26: 143-151. doi: 10.7555/JBR.26.20120027.

He, L., Liu, B., Xipeng, G., Xie, G., Liao, S., Quan, D., Chai, D., Lu, J., & Ramakrishna, S. 2009. "Microstructure and properties of nano-fibrous PCL-b-PLLA scaffolds for cartilage tissue engineering." *Eur Cell Mater*, 18: 63-74. URL: http://citeseerx.ist.psu.edu/viewdoc/download?doi=10.1.1.460.7280&rep=rep1&type=pdf.

Husain, S., Al-Samadani, K. H., Najeeb, S., Zafar, M. S., Khurshid, Z., Zohaib, S., & Qasim, S. B. 2017. "Chitosan biomaterials for current and potential dental applications." *Materials*, 10: 602. doi: 10.3390/ma10060602.

Jorio, A. (Ed.). 2016. *Bioengineering applications of carbon nanostructures*. Springer International Publishing. doi: 10.1007%2F978-3-319-25907-9.

Keller, L., Offner, D., Schwinté, P., Morand, D., Wagner, Q., Gros, C., Bornert, F., Bahi, S., Musset, A. N., Jessel, N. B., & Fioretti, F. 2015. "Active nanomaterials to meet the challenge of dental pulp regeneration." *Materials*, 8: 7461-7471. doi: 10.3390/ma8115387.

Khetawat, S., & Lodha, S. 2015. "Nanotechnology (nanohydroxyapatite crystals): recent advancement in treatment of dentinal hyper-sensitivity." *J Interdiscipl Med Dent Sci*, 3: 181. doi: 10.4172/ 2376032X.1000181.

Khurshid, Z., Zafar, M., Qasim, S., Shahab, S., Naseem, M., & AbuReqaiba, A. 2015. "Advances in nanotechnology for restorative dentistry." *Materials*, 8: 717-731. doi: 10.3390/ma8020717.

Lboutounne, H. 2017. "Dental Medicine Nanosystems: Nanoparticles and their use in Dentistry and Oral Health Care." *Int J Dent & Oral Heal*, 3: 145-157. doi: 10.25141/2471-657X-2017-10.0150.

Martins-Júnior, P. A., Alcântara, C. E., Resende, R. R., & Ferreira, A. J. 2013. "Carbon nanotubes: directions and perspectives in oral regenerative medicine." *Journal of dental research*, 92: 575-583. doi: 10.1177/0022034513490957.

McIntyre, R. A. 2012. "Common nano-materials and their use in real world applications." *Science progress*, 95: 1-22. URL: https://europepmc.org/abstract/MED/22574383.

Monteiro, D. R., Gorup, L. F., Takamiya, A. S., de Camargo, E. R., Filho, A. C. R., & Barbosa, D. B. 2012. "Silver distribution and release from an antimicrobial denture base resin containing silver colloidal nanoparticles." *Journal of Prosthodontics: Implant, Esthetic and Reconstructive Dentistry*, 21: 7-15. doi: 10.1111/j.1532-849X.2011.00772.x.

Moradkhani, M. R., Karimi, A., & Negahdari, B. 2018. "Nanotechnology application to local anaesthesia (LA)." *Artificial cells, nanomedicine, and biotechnology*, 46: 355-360. doi: 10.1080/21691401.2017.1313263.

Neel, E. A. A., Bozec, L., Perez, R. A., Kim, H. W., & Knowles, J. C. 2015. "Nanotechnology in dentistry: prevention, diagnosis, and therapy." *International journal of nanomedicine*, 10: 6371-6394. doi: 10.2147/IJN.S86033.

Pachauri, P., Bathala, L. R., & Sangur, R. 2014. "Techniques for dental implant nanosurface modifications." *The journal of advanced prosthodontics*, 6: 498-504. doi: 10.4047/jap.2014.6.6.498.

Persson, C., Unosson, E., Ajaxon, I., Engstrand, J., Engqvist, H., & Xia, W. 2012. "Nano grain sized zirconia–silica glass ceramics for dental applications." *Journal of the European Ceramic Society*, 32: 4105-4110. doi : 10.1016/j.jeurceramsoc.2012.06.028.

Popovtzer, R., Agrawal, A., Kotov, N. A., Popovtzer, A., Balter, J., Carey, T. E., & Kopelman, R. 2008. "Targeted gold nanoparticles enable molecular CT imaging of cancer." *Nano letters*, 8: 4593-4596. doi: 10.1021/nl8029114.

Priyadarsini, S., Mukherjee, S., & Mishra, M. 2018. "Nanoparticles used in dentistry: A review." *Journal of oral biology and craniofacial research*, 8: 58-67. doi: 10.1016/j.jobcr.2017.12.004.

Riquieri, H., Monteiro, J. B., Viegas, D. C., Campos, T. M. B., de Melo, R. M., & Saavedra, G. D. S. F. A. 2018. "Impact of crystallization firing process on the microstructure and flexural strength of zirconia-reinforced lithium silicate glass-ceramics." *Dental Materials*, 34: 1483-1491. doi: 10.1016/j.dental.2018.06.010.

Rogers, J. A. 2015. "Electronics for the human body." *Jama*, 313: 561-562. doi: 10.1001/jama.2014.17915.

Sachdeva, S., Kapoor, P., Tamrakar, A. K., & Noor, R. 2015. "Nano-composite dental resins: an overview." *Annals of Dental Specialty*, 3: 52-55. URL: https://pdfs.semanticscholar.org/714a/35db214c61155 cb4e37fa9050e9f3f5c2129.pdf.

Salata, O. V. 2004. "Applications of nanoparticles in biology and medicine." *Journal of nanobiotechnology*, 2: 3. doi: 10.1186/1477-3155-2-3.

Santamaria, C. M., Woodruff, A., Yang, R., & Kohane, D. S. 2017. "Drug delivery systems for prolonged duration local anesthesia." *Materials Today*, 20: 22-31. doi : 10.1016/j.mattod.2016.11.019.

Shakib, K., Tan, A., Soskic, V., & Seifalian, A. M. 2014. "Regenerative nanotechnology in oral and maxillofacial surgery." *British Journal of Oral and Maxillofacial Surgery*, 52: 884-893. doi: 10.1016/j.bjoms. 2014.08.006.

Tomsia, A. P., Lee, J. S., Wegst, U. G. K., Saiz E. 2013. "Nanotechnology for dental implants." *Int J Oral Maxillofac Implants* 28.

Xie, H., Cao, T., Rodríguez-Lozano, F. J., Luong-Van, E. K., & Rosa, V. 2017. "Graphene for the development of the next-generation of biocomposites for dental and medical applications." *Dental Materials*, 33: 765-774. doi: 10.1016/j.dental.2017.04.008.

Yeh, C. K., Christodoulides, N. J., Floriano, P. N., Miller, C. S., Ebersole, J. L., Weigum, S. E., Devitt, J., & Redding, S. W. 2010. "Current development of saliva/oral fluid-based diagnostics." *Texas dental journal*, 127: 651. URL: https://www.ncbi.nlm.nih.gov/pmc/articles/ PMC3742318/.

Zhou, H., & Lee, J. 2011. "Nanoscale hydroxyapatite particles for bone tissue engineering." *Acta biomaterialia*, 7: 2769-2781. doi: 10.1016/j.actbio.2011.03.019.

ABOUT THE EDITORS

Dr. Aneeya Kumar Samantara
School of Chemical Sciences
National Institute of Science Education and Research
Bhubaneswar, Odisha, India

Dr. Aneeya Kumar Samantara is a post-doctorate fellow at National Institute of Science Education and Research, Odisha, India. He did his Ph.D. in Chemistry from CSIR-Institute of Minerals and Materials Technology, Odisha, India. Before joining Ph.D., he completed Master in Science in Advanced Organic Chemistry from Ravenshaw University, and Master of philosophy (M.Phil.) from Utkal University. Aneeya's research interest includes the development different metal/non-metal nanostructures for energy storage/conversion, sensing and biomedical applications. To his credit, he has authored in 22 peer reviewed international journals, Nine Books and four book chapters. To his credits he has been awarded in many National and International Forums.

Dr. Satyajit Ratha
School of Basic Sciences
National Institute of Science Education and Research
Bhubaneswar, Odisha, India

Dr. Satyajit Ratha has pursued his Ph.D. at the Indian Institute of Technology Bhubaneswar, India. Prior to joining IIT Bhubaneswar, he received his Bachelor of Science, First Class Honours from Utkal University, in 2008 and Master of Science from Ravenshaw University in 2010. Satyajit's research interests include two dimensional semiconductors, nanostructure synthesis, applications, energy storage devices and supercapacitors. He has authored and co-authored about 21 peer reviewed international journals, Six Books and one Book Chapter.

INDEX

B

D

E

I

K

L

M

O

P

Q

R

S

T

U

V

Related Nova Publications

Mechanical Ventilation: Applications, Technologies and Ethical Issues

Editor: Antonio M. Esquinas

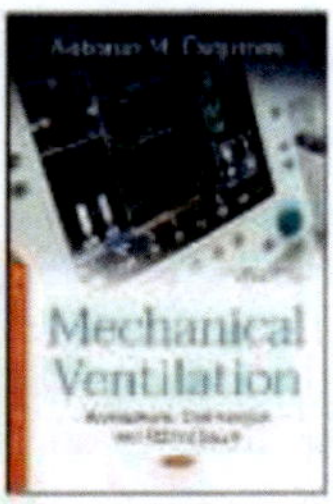

Series: Advances in Respiratory and Critical Care Medicine

Book Description: This book has made a selection of the hot topics about indications of mechanical ventilation, technological development advances, ethical and cost associated with mechanical ventilation.

Hardcover ISBN: 978-1-53615-002-5
Retail Price: $230

Advances in Radiometry Research

Author: Perry Xiao, Ph.D.

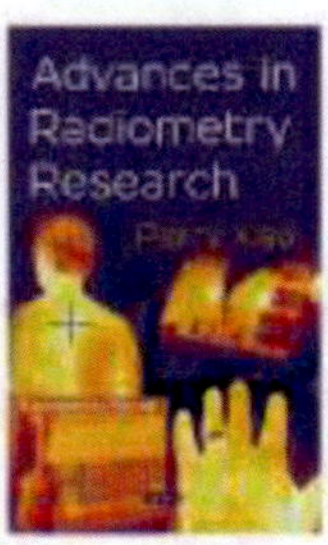

Series: Biomedical Devices and their Applications

Book Description: Radiometry is a fascinating, fast growing research area, and there are many interesting real life applications. This book is intended to provide readers the theoretical background of radiometry, a resource of the latest radiometry technology, as well as the latest research in radiometry.

Hardcover ISBN: 978-1-53614-726-1
Retail Price: $230

To see a complete list of Nova publications, please visit our website at www.novapublishers.com